Balloon-Assisted Enteroscopy

Jong-Jae Park • Hironori Yamamoto
Hyun Joo Jang • Sung Noh Hong
Editors

Balloon-Assisted Enteroscopy

Springer

Editors
Jong-Jae Park
Division of Gastroenterology, Department of Internal Medicine
Korea University College of Medicine
Seoul, Korea (Republic of)

Hironori Yamamoto
Department of Medicine, Division of Gastroenterology
Jichi Medical University
Shimotsuke, Tochigi, Japan

Hyun Joo Jang
Department of Gastroenterology
Hallym University School of Medicine
Hwaseong, Kyonggi-do, Korea (Republic of)

Sung Noh Hong
Department of Medicine
Samsung Medical Center, Sungkyunkwan University School of Medicine
Seoul, Korea (Republic of)

ISBN 978-981-95-2444-0 ISBN 978-981-95-2445-7 (eBook)
https://doi.org/10.1007/978-981-95-2445-7

English translation of the 1st original Korean edition published by SnC Publishing, Seoul, 2021

Translation from the Korean language edition: "Balloon-Assisted Enteroscopy" by Jong-Jae Park et al.,

This Springer imprint is published by the registered company Springer Nature Singapore Pte Ltd.
The registered company address is: 152 Beach Road, #21-01/04 Gateway East, Singapore 189721, Singapore

Preface

Since its introduction in the early 2000s, balloon-assisted enteroscopy (BAE) has revolutionized the diagnosis and management of small bowel diseases. As one of the most advanced techniques in gastrointestinal endoscopy, BAE continues to evolve with innovations in device technology and procedural expertise.

This textbook was conceived to provide a comprehensive, practical, and up-to-date reference for clinicians, trainees, and researchers involved in BAE. It covers the full spectrum of BAE—from fundamental principles and techniques to cutting-edge therapeutic applications—with contributions from leading experts in the field.

The Korean Society of Gastrointestinal Endoscopy (KSGE), as a long-standing academic society dedicated to the advancement of gastrointestinal endoscopy, is proud to support the publication of this book. KSGE has played a pivotal role in research and education in the field of gastrointestinal endoscopy, both in Korea and internationally. This textbook reflects our ongoing commitment to promoting excellence in endoscopic practice.

I would like to express my sincere appreciation to the editorial team, contributing authors, and all those who have supported this endeavor. I hope that this contribution will serve as a valuable guide and inspiration for current and future generations of endoscopists.

Seoul, South Korea — Jong-Jae Park
Tochigi, Japan — Hironori Yamamoto
Hwaseong, South Korea — Hyun Joo Jang
Seoul, South Korea — Sung Noh Hong

Acknowledgments

I would like to convey my deepest gratitude to all the authors who contributed their invaluable time and expertise to this textbook, amid the intensified clinical burdens arising from the unprecedented challenges within the Korean healthcare system, particularly affecting referral hospitals and tertiary care institutions. Their unwavering commitment to excellence in clinical practice and education was essential to completing each chapter.

Special acknowledgment and sincere appreciation are due to Professor Hironori Yamamoto of Jichi Medical University in Japan, the inventor of double-balloon enteroscopy. His pioneering work in 2001 laid the fundamental scientific groundwork upon which this volume is based.

Furthermore, I am profoundly grateful to the Research Group for Capsule Endoscopy and Enteroscopy of the Korean Society of Gastrointestinal Endoscopy. The dedicated leadership and diligent efforts of both past and present chairs and members of the group have significantly fostered a collaborative and enriching academic environment essential to this project.

Since its establishment as the Gut Image Study Group in August 2004, the research group has consistently made substantial contributions through multicenter studies, annual symposia, educational workshops, and the creation of a comprehensive database. Collectively, their efforts have greatly advanced the field of small-bowel endoscopy. This textbook stands as a tribute to their remarkable achievements and continued dedication.

Department of Medicine, Samsung Medical Center
Sungkyunkwan University School of Medicine
Seoul, South Korea

Sung Noh Hong

Research Group for Capsule Endoscopy and Enteroscopy
Korean Society of Gastrointestinal Endoscopy
Seoul, South Korea

Contents

Editors and Contributors

Editors

Jong-Jae Park Division of Gastroenterology, Department of Internal Medicine, Korea University Guro Hospital, Korea University College of Medicine, Seoul, South Korea

Hironori Yamamoto Department of Medicine, Division of Gastroenterology, Jichi Medical University, Tochigi, Japan

Hyun Joo Jang Department of Gastroenterology, Hallym University Dongtan Sacred Heart Hospital, Hallym University School of Medicine, Hwaseong, South Korea

Sung Noh Hong Department of Medicine, Samsung Medical Center, Sungkyunkwan University School of Medicine, Seoul, South Korea

Contributors

Hwang Choi College of Medicine, The Catholic University of Korea, Incheon, South Korea

Chang Soo Eun College of Medicine, Hanyang University, Guri, South Korea

Seung Min Hong Pusan National University College of Medicine, Pusan, South Korea

Sung Noh Hong Sungkyunkwan University School of Medicine, Seoul, South Korea

Hyun Joo Jang Hallym University School of Medicine, Dongtan, South Korea

Seong Ran Jeon Soonchunhyang University College of Medicine, Seoul, South Korea

Eun Ran Kim Sungkyunkwan University School of Medicine, Seoul, South Korea

Jinsu Kim College of Medicine, The Catholic University of Korea, Seoul, South Korea

Bong Min Ko Soonchunhyang University College of Medicine, Bucheon, South Korea

Beom Jae Lee Korea University College of Medicine, Seoul, South Korea

Hyunjung Lee Seoul National University College of Medicine, Seoul, South Korea

Jae Gon Lee Hallym University School of Medicine, Dongtan, South Korea

Jae Joon Park Yonsei University College of Medicine, Seoul, South Korea

Ye Hyun Park Ewha Womans University School of Medicine, Seoul, South Korea

Satoshi Shinozaki Jichi Medical University, Tochigi, Japan

Hironori Yamamoto Jichi Medical University, Tochigi, Japan

Dong-Hoon Yang University of Ulsan College of Medicine, Seoul, South Korea

Tomonori Yano Jichi Medical University, Tochigi, Japan

Overview of Small Bowel Enteroscopy

1

Seung Min Hong, Hwang Choi, Chang Soo Eun,
Beom Jae Lee, Jae Gon Lee, and Hyun Joo Jang

1.1 History of Small Bowel Enteroscopy

1.1.1 Introduction

The small bowel, approximately 6 m in length, poses limitations for endoscopic examination. While upper gastrointestinal endoscopy can reach the duodenum and colonoscopy can view the terminal ileum, most of the small bowel remains inaccessible. Traditional methods of small bowel enteroscopy—such as push, sonde, and ropeway techniques—have been used but allow only partial visualization of the jejunum. These methods are difficult to perform and often cause considerable discomfort for patients, limiting their broader application. In the twenty-first century, capsule endoscopy and balloon-assisted enteroscopy have enabled complete examination of the small bowel, facilitating accurate diagnosis and endoscopic treatment

S. M. Hong
Pusan National University School of Medicine, Yangsan, South Korea
e-mail: lucky77i@naver.com

H. Choi (✉)
College of Medicine, The Catholic University of Korea, Seoul, South Korea
e-mail: hwchoi@catholic.ac.kr

C. S. Eun
Hanyang University College of Medicine, Seoul, South Korea
e-mail: cseun@hanyang.ac.kr

B. J. Lee
Division of Gastroenterology, Korea University College of Medicine, Seoul, South Korea
e-mail: L85210@korea.ac.kr

J. G. Lee · H. J. Jang
Hallym University Dongtan Sacred Heart Hospital, Gyeonggi, South Korea
e-mail: jhj1229@hallym.or.kr

J.-J. Park et al. (eds.), *Balloon-Assisted Enteroscopy*,
https://doi.org/10.1007/978-981-95-2445-7_1

of small bowel diseases. Examining the development and history of small bowel enteroscopy can deepen the understanding of this technique and highlight potential future advancements.

1.1.2 History of Small Bowel Enteroscopy

Since the development of the gastrocamera and fiberscope in the 1950s, various techniques have been explored for observing the small bowel (Fig. 1.1).

In Japan in 1971, Hiratsuka was the first to attempt the ropeway method of small bowel enteroscopy, followed by Classen in Germany in 1972 (Table 1.1) [1, 2]. This method used a 2-m-long fiberscope inserted over a thin Teflon tube prepositioned in the distal ileum to visualize the small bowel. Classen successfully advanced the scope to the distal ileum in 8 of 10 patients, diagnosing 1 case of jejunoileitis with multiple ulcers and polypoid lesions. However, this method was eventually abandoned due to the procedural difficulty and significant discomfort it caused for patients.

The ropeway method for small bowel enteroscopy was initially reported in 1982. Using the Olympus SIF-M (Olympus, Tokyo, Japan), Tada et al. [2, 3] conducted small bowel enteroscopy in 11 patients, diagnosing 3 cases of ileal tuberculosis and Crohn's disease through magnifying lens and biopsy.

The development of the sonde small bowel enteroscopy began in 1974, progressing through various prototypes that included either a balloon at the end of the enteroscope or a flexible tip [2–4]. The Olympus SSIF type VII (Olympus, Tokyo, Japan), introduced in 1986, featured a narrow 5-mm tip that allowed for nasal insertion.

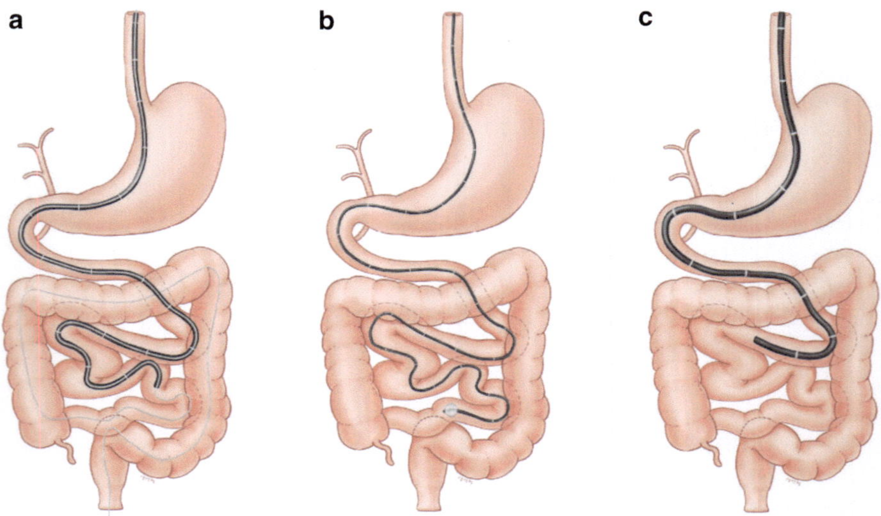

Fig. 1.1 Methods of small bowel enteroscopy in the past. (**a**) Ropeway technique. (**b**) Sonde technique. (**c**) Push technique

Table 1.1 History of the small bowel enteroscopy

Insertion method	Product name	Manufacturer	Reporter	Year
Ropeway	–	–	Hiratsuka H [1]	1971
Ropeway	JF-D	Olympus	Classen M [2]	1972
Ropeway	SIF-M	Olympus	Tada M [2]	1982
Sonde	SSIF type VII	Olympus	Tada M [2]	1986
Sonde	SIF VI KAI	Olympus	Gostout CJ [4]	1991
Sonde	ESI-2000	Pentax	Dabezies MA [2]	1991
Sonde	SIF-SW	Olympus	Morris AJ [2]	1992
Push	SIF-B	Olympus	Ogoshi K [2, 3]	1973
Push	SIF-10 L	Olympus	Shimizu S [5]	1987
Push	SIF-100	Olympus	Barkin JS [2]	1994
Push	VSB-P2900	Pentax	Dykman DD [2]	1993
Push	SIF-140Q	Olympus	Benz C [10]	2002
Double balloon	EN-450P5/20	Fujinon	Yamamoto H [7]	2001
Single balloon	SIF-Q180/Q260	Olympus	Kawamura T [10]	2007
Spiral	Endo-ease	Spirus	Akerman PA [9]	2007
Spiral	PowerSpiral	Olympus	Neuhaus H [8]	2015

Although this model reduced patient's discomfort compared to earlier oral sonde enteroscopes, its use is limited as it did not permit biopsy or therapeutic procedures.

In 1991, a 4-m-long video sonde small bowel enteroscope (ESI-2000; Pentax, New York, USA) was developed alongside the SIF VI KAI (Olympus, Tokyo, Japan), an oral sonde small bowel enteroscope featuring a 12-mm tip that enabled biopsy and four-way flexion [2]. Among 35 patients with unexplained gastrointestinal bleeding, the enteroscope reached the terminal ileum in 14% of cases, the mid to distal ileum in 69%, and the jejunum in 17%. Abnormal findings, primarily vascular anomalies of the mucosa, were identified in 26% of these patients [4].

In 1973, push-type small bowel enteroscopy was performed in Japan to obtain suction biopsies from the proximal jejunum for enzyme analysis and microscopic examination [2]. The SIF-B (Olympus, Tokyo, Japan), with a 10-mm tip and a working length of 1620 mm, was inserted 30 cm past the ligament of Treitz. In the 1980s, both adult and pediatric colonoscopes were used orally to examine the jejunum up to approximately 50 cm below the ligament of Treitz. A push-type small bowel enteroscope (SIF-10 L; Olympus Tokyo, Japan) with a 2175-mm working length and an overtube extended insertion depth to 60–120 cm [5]. In the early 1990s introduction of the 2500-mm-long video Pentax small bowel enteroscope (VSB-P2900; Pentax, New York, USA) and Olympus small bowel enteroscope (SIF-100; Olympus, Tokyo, Japan), push-type small bowel enteroscopy became an effective clinical tool for diagnosing suspected small bowel diseases, including cases of unexplained gastrointestinal bleeding [2].

1.1.3 Current State of Small Bowel Enteroscopy

In the twenty-first century, advancements in smart technology and imaging have brought significant progress to small bowel enteroscopy, ushering in a revolutionary period for the field. While several techniques exist for examining the small bowel, their widespread adoption has been limited by certain constraints. With the advent of capsule endoscopy, diagnosing small bowel diseases has become safer and more comfortable, while balloon-assisted enteroscopy, using balloons and an overtube, has enabled both diagnosis and treatment through endoscopy [6, 7]. Improved radiological imaging techniques now offer enhanced imaging and more accurate diagnoses than previous methods. These two methods currently play complementary roles in small bowel examination.

Capsule endoscopy was originally developed for military purposes in Israel. In 2000, the M2A capsule (Given Imaging, Yokneam, Israel) was first used for patients with unexplained gastrointestinal bleeding and received approval for use in the United States and Europe in 2001. Following this, esophageal and colon capsule endoscopes were introduced, and small bowel capsule endoscopy saw continuous improvements, from the PillCam SB1 (Medtronic, Minneapolis, MN, USA) to the SB3. Other capsule endoscopes, such as the MiroCam (IntroMedic, Seoul, Korea) and ENDOCAPSULE (Olympus, Tokyo, Japan), were also released. A Binocular Capsule Endoscope (IntroMedic, Seoul, Korea) capable of capturing 3D stereoscopic images with two cameras was developed. Additionally, the CapsoCam Plus SV-3 (CapsoVision Inc., Saratoga, CA, USA), a capsule endoscope with four side cameras providing a 360° panoramic view, was introduced.

Double-balloon enteroscopy, which uses a balloon at the end of a 2-m-long enteroscope and another at the distal end of the overtube, makes it significantly easier to examine the entire small bowel compared to previous sonde or push-type small bowel enteroscopies. This technique was first introduced by Yamamoto in 2001 using a Fujinon small bowel enteroscope (EN-450P5/20; Fujinon Corp., Saitama, Japan) [1, 7]. In sonde small bowel enteroscopy, the balloon aids deep insertion by enhancing peristalsis, while in push-type enteroscopy, the overtube helps straighten the endoscope in the stomach and duodenum. In double-balloon

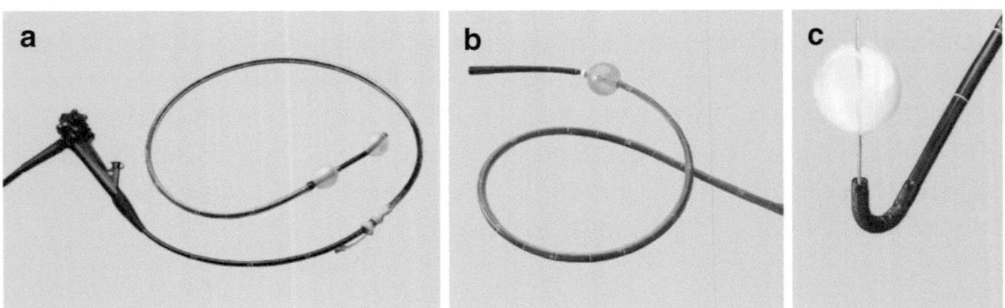

Fig. 1.2 Balloon-assisted enteroscope. (**a**) Double-balloon enteroscope. (**b**) Single-balloon enteroscope. (**c**) Balloon-guided enteroscope

enteroscopy, the combined use of the balloons and overtube maximizes the effect of shortening the small bowel. Furthermore, therapeutic enteroscopes (EN-450 T5, EN-580 T; Fujinon Corp, Saitama, Japan) with larger forceps channels (2.8–3.2 mm, compared to the previous 2.2 mm) were developed (Fig. 1.2), enabling a wide range of enteroscopic procedures, including hemostasis, tumor resection, dilation, and foreign body removal in the small bowel.

Single-balloon enteroscopy, introduced by Olympus in 2007 (SIF-Q260; Olympus, Tokyo, Japan), uses a 2-m-long enteroscope with a balloon only on the overtube, not at the end [8, 9]. While it offers slightly less coverage of the small bowel compared to double-balloon enteroscopy, it remains effective for diagnosing and treating small bowel diseases.

Since then, various device-assisted enteroscopy methods have been developed [8–10]. Balloon-guided endoscopy (NaviAidTM AB; Smart Medical, Ra'anana, Israel), introduced in 2008, is conceptually the opposite of single-balloon enteroscopy. It involves inserting a 3.5-m-long catheter with a 40-mm balloon through the existing enteroscope working channel to examine the small bowel (Fig. 1.2). Spiral enteroscopy, developed in 2007, employs a different insertion method. It uses a manually rotatable Endo-Ease overtube (Spirus Medical, West Bridgewater, MA, USA) attached to a balloon-assisted small bowel enteroscope or pediatric colonoscope (Fig. 1.3). Initial reports mentioned mucosal damage, but improvements in the spiral overtube have minimized these effects. This method is typically performed orally and requires an assistant endoscopist to help adjust the overtube for smooth insertion. In 2015, PowerSpiral Motorized Enteroscopy (Olympus, Tokyo, Japan) was developed, which is powered by a foot pedal, making insertion easier and reducing the time required.

In Korea, capsule endoscopy has been used clinically since 2002, followed by the introduction of double-balloon enteroscopy in 2004 and single-balloon enteroscopy in 2008.

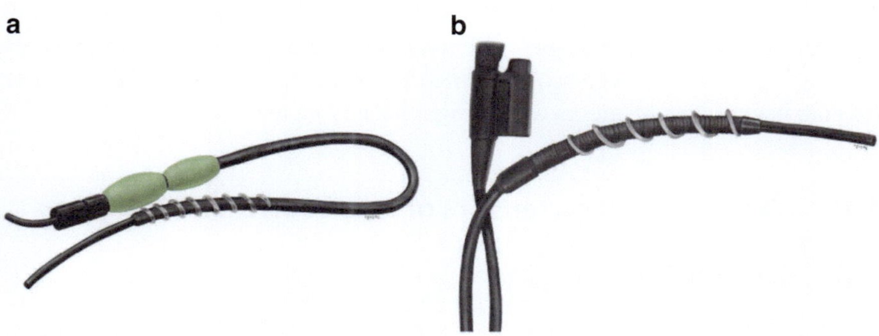

Fig. 1.3 Spiral enteroscope. (**a**) Manual spiral enteroscope. (**b**) Automated spiral enteroscope

Table 1.2 Use of overtube and balloon in small bowel enteroscopy

Insertion method	Product name	Total length, mm	Tip diameter, mm	Channel diameter, mm	Overtube	Balloon
Ropeway	SIF-M	2010	11.0	2.8	–	–
	SIF-2C	1900	11.0	2.8/2.0	–	–
	JF-D	3000	10.0	2.8	–	–
	SIF-RP	1625	11.0	2.8	–	–
Sonde	SSIF type VII	3010	5.4	–	–	Optional
	SIF VI KAI	2675	12.0	2.0	–	Optional
	ESI-2000	4000	12.5	–	–	–
	SIF-SW	3000	5.4	1.0/1.0	–	Optional
Push	SIF-B	1770	10.0	2.8	–	–
	SIF-10 L	2495	11.2	2.8	Optional	–
	SIF-100	2500	11.2	2.8	Optional	–
	VSB-3430 K	2200	11.6	3.8	–	–
	SIF-140Q	2500	10.5	2.8	Optional	–
Double balloon	EN-450P5/20	2300	8.5	2.2	Mandatory	Mandatory
	EN-450 T5	2300	9.4	2.8	Mandatory	Mandatory
	EN-580XP	2300	7.5	2.2	Mandatory	Mandatory
	EN-580 T	2300	9.4	3.2	Mandatory	Mandatory
	EI-580BT	1850	9.4	3.2	Mandatory	Mandatory
Single balloon	SIF-Q180/ Q260	2345	9.2	2.8	Mandatory	Mandatory
	SIF-H290S	1830	9.2	3.2	Mandatory	Mandatory
Spiral	Endo-ease	–	14.5	9.8	Mandatory	–
	PSF-1	2015	11.2	3.2	–	–

1.1.4 Future of Small Bowel Enteroscopy

Over the past 50 years, various methods for visualizing and treating the small bowel have been developed. While balloons attached to the endoscope tip or overtube have been used to reach the deeper parts of the small bowel, the advancement of device-assisted enteroscopy using balloons and overtubes has made both the diagnosis and the treatment of small bowel conditions easier and more accurate (Table 1.2). Looking ahead, new technologies will continue to emerge, aiming to improve the safety of small bowel enteroscopy, shorten procedure times, and enhance comfort for both patients and operators without significantly increasing costs.

1.2 Types and Characteristics of Small Bowel Enteroscopy

1.2.1 Introduction

Endoscopic access to the small bowel has been challenging due to its distant location from both the mouth and the anus. In the early 2000s, capsule endoscopy (CE)

and double-balloon enteroscopy (DBE) were introduced, enabling full observation of the small bowel, and significantly advancing the diagnosis and treatment of small bowel diseases. While CE offers a painless method for observing the entire small bowel, it cannot perform biopsies or therapeutic procedures, is time-consuming to review, and cannot pinpoint the exact location of the lesions. Small bowel enteroscopy, though more invasive, allows for real-time observation and the ability to perform biopsies and therapies. Currently, the types of enteroscopy used in clinical practice include device-assisted enteroscopy, push enteroscopy, and intraoperative enteroscopy, with device-assisted enteroscopy including DBE, single-balloon enteroscopy (SBE), and spiral enteroscopy. This chapter provides an overview of the different types and characteristics of small bowel enteroscopy.

1.2.2 Double-Balloon Enteroscopy

DBE, developed to examine the entire small bowel, was introduced in 2001. It involves a specially designed enteroscope and overtube, each with a latex balloon at the distal end, along with a balloon pump system to control the inflation and deflation of the balloons. The balloon on the overtube tip anchors the small bowel, preventing excessive extension when advancing the scope, thus facilitating insertion. Once the small bowel is anchored, the overtube is advanced and pulled to pleat and shorten the bowel, enabling the scope to reach deeper sections of the small bowel [11].

DBE allows for endoscopic evaluation of the entire small bowel either through a single approach or by combining antegrade and retrograde methods. It also enables tissue biopsy and therapeutic interventions. The mean procedure time ranges from 73 to 123 min, with an insertion depth of 220–360 cm for the antegrade approach, and 124–183 cm for the retrograde approach. The diagnostic yield for clinically significant small bowel diseases is comparable to CE (60% vs. 57%) [12].

However, DBE requires skill and the presence of two operators. Its drawbacks include longer procedure time, fewer complications, but more invasive, uncomfortable for the patient, and labor-intensive for the operator. Typically, performing both antegrade and retrograde approaches on the same day is not recommended.

1.2.3 Single-Balloon Enteroscopy

SBE, introduced in 2007, consists of an enteroscope, an overtube, and a balloon pump system to control the inflation and deflation of the balloon. Unlike DBE, SBE does not have a balloon at the tip of the enteroscope; instead, a silicone balloon is mounted at the distal end of the overtube. The insertion method is similar to DBE, but simpler, as it does not involve manipulating a balloon on the enteroscope. The enteroscope is advanced, the tip is flexed and hooked into the small bowel folds to prevent slippage, the overtube is advanced, and the balloon on the overtube is inflated and fixed to the bowel wall. Both the scope and overtube are pulled to shorten the small bowel, allowing the enteroscope to be advanced into the deeper parts of the small bowel [13].

SBE is easier to learn and simpler to perform than DBE, and it can be carried out by a single operator without the need for an assistant. The preparation time is also shorter since there is no balloon at the tip of the enteroscope. SBE has diagnostic yields of 41–65% and therapeutic yields of 7–50%, similar to DBE. However, due to the absence of balloon anchoring at the tip of the enteroscope, it is more challenging to examine the deep small bowel and has a lower rate of complete small bowel evaluation compared to DBE. The mean insertion depth for SBE is reported to be 133–270 cm for the antegrade approach and 73–199 cm for the retrograde approach [12].

1.2.4 Spiral Enteroscopy

Spiral enteroscopy, introduced in 2007, features a 5.5-mm high spiral helix at the distal end of the overtube, which resembles a screwdriver, allowing for easier and faster insertion compared to conventional balloon-assisted enteroscopy. When the overtube is attached to the enteroscope and the overtube is rotated clockwise, the small bowel is pleated around the overtube as the scope advances. When the scope is withdrawn for observation, the overtube is rotated counterclockwise.

Manual spiral enteroscopy was replaced by motorized spiral enteroscopy, which was introduced in 2016. This system features an electric motor controlled by the operator, located in the enteroscope's handle to rotate the spiral overtube. The rotation, both clockwise and counterclockwise, is controlled via a foot pedal [14]. While large studies have shown promising results regarding efficacy, procedure time and pan-enteroscopy rates, safety concerns have arisen. As a result, motorized spiral enteroscopy was withdrawn from the global market in July 2023 due to several serious adverse events and is no longer available in clinical practice [15].

1.2.5 Push Enteroscopy

Push enteroscopy is a method for examining the small bowel using a specialized enteroscope or colonoscope that is inserted through the mouth. The scope is advanced as far as possible until it encounters a loop, usually reaching the proximal jejunum. An overtube is usually not used due to patient's discomfort and reported adverse events associated with its use.

Push enteroscopy is commonly used to examine small bowel lesions up to the proximal jejunum, as it is simple and widely available and does not require special equipment or training. The insertion depth is typically around 45–60 cm beyond the ligament of Treitz with a colonoscope, and the diagnostic yield for obscure gastrointestinal bleeding ranges from 15% to 40% [16].

1.2.6 Intraoperative Enteroscopy

Intraoperative enteroscopy involves inserting an enteroscope orally or through an enterotomy in the operating room to examine the deep small bowel with surgical assistance. The surgeon uses a laparotomy or laparoscopic technique to pleat the small bowel over the enteroscope, enabling the endoscopist to inspect the small bowel and either treat the lesion endoscopically or mark it for surgical resection.

This method is the most invasive enteroscopic approach, but provides a comprehensive evaluation of the entire small bowel. However, intraoperative enteroscopy is time-consuming, requiring the efforts of the surgical team, endoscopist, and other resources, and has a high complication rate. Due to advances in noninvasive imaging and device-assisted enteroscopy, it is now rarely used and requires careful patient selection.

1.3 Indications, Advantages, and Contraindications of Balloon-Assisted Enteroscopy

1.3.1 Introduction

The diagnosis and treatment of small-bowel lesions underwent a significant shift after the development of capsule endoscopy in 2000 and Fujinon's double-balloon enteroscopy (DBE) in 2001. With these advancements, although previously considered difficult within the field of gastroenterology, diagnostic and therapeutic approaches to the small bowel have become feasible. Subsequently, Olympus developed single-balloon enteroscopy (SBE), which has been applied in clinical practice. The development of these balloon-assisted enteroscopy techniques has resulted in

Table 1.3 Indications of balloon-assisted enteroscopy

Indications	Procedures
Small-bowel bleeding	Hemostasis (argon plasma and clipping)
Malignant tumors of the small bowel	Biopsy, preoperative marking, stent placement
Crohn's disease	Biopsy and balloon dilation
Small-bowel inflammatory diseases and strictures (e.g., celiac disease, NSAID-induced enteropathy)	Biopsy and balloon dilation
Polyposis syndromes (e.g., familial adenomatous polyposis, Peutz-Jeghers syndrome)	Polypectomy
Small-bowel obstruction caused by foreign bodies	Foreign body removal
Patients with roux-en-Y anastomosis	ERCP, therapeutic endoscopy
Patients with difficulties undergoing colonoscopy	Colonoscopy, therapeutic endoscopy
Others	Percutaneous endoscopic jejunostomy placement

NSAID nonsteroidal anti-inflammatory drugs

real-time observation, biopsy, and therapeutic procedures for small-bowel lesions, leading to rapid advancements in the understanding and research of small-bowel diseases. However, enteroscopy should be performed by highly skilled endoscopists. This is because the procedure typically takes >1 hour and it may involve radiation exposure to validate entry. Hence, it is not considered in routine endoscopic examination. This section aimed to examine the indications, advantages, and contraindications of balloon-assisted enteroscopy [17–24].

1.3.2 Indications (Table 1.3)

1.3.2.1 Small-Bowel Bleeding Lesions

Small-bowel bleeding lesion is the most common indication of balloon-assisted enteroscopy. With the increasing use of non-steroidal anti-inflammatory drugs and antiplatelet agents, the incidence of bleeding disorders in the small bowel has increased, leading to the more frequent use of balloon-assisted enteroscopy. The procedure is performed if there is bleeding of unknown source on upper gastrointestinal or colonoscopy examinations, which suggests small-bowel bleeding. Further, balloon-assisted enteroscopy can be conducted independently or in combination with capsule endoscopy. Hemostasis can be performed during diagnosis if the patient's vital signs are stable.

1.3.2.2 Tumorous Lesions in the Small Bowel

If imaging tests such as capsule endoscopy and abdominal computed tomography scan can detect tumorous lesions, balloon-assisted enteroscopy may be conducted for presurgical biopsy. This method is valuable for marking small submucosal tumors, such as neuroendocrine tumors, which are challenging to identify during surgery. Balloon-assisted enteroscopy is also used in diagnosing and treating polyps associated with genetic conditions such as familial adenomatous polyposis and Peutz-Jeghers syndrome. Notably, polypectomy helps avoid surgical bowel resection in patients with Peutz-Jeghers syndrome.

1.3.2.3 Crohn's Disease

In patients suspected of or diagnosed with Crohn's disease, balloon-assisted enteroscopy can be performed for biopsy to validate diagnosis, assess treatment response, and provide therapeutic balloon dilation for accompanying strictures.

1.3.2.4 Diagnosis and Treatment of Small-Bowel Strictures/Obstruction

Balloon-assisted enteroscopy allows the performance of biopsy to distinguish benign from malignant strictures that do not involve necrosis. For short strictures, balloon dilation can be performed, and stenting can be considered to relieve symptoms in cases of malignant obstruction.

1.3.2.5 Foreign Body Removal

Although rare, balloon-assisted enteroscopy can be used to remove foreign objects from the small bowel. For example, retained capsules caused by stricture during diagnostic procedures or displaced gastrointestinal stents causing obstructions can be removed without surgery. Previous reports have shown that the success rate of this technique for foreign body removal is approximately 50%.

1.3.2.6 Differentiation of Inflammatory Diseases

Balloon-assisted enteroscopy may be used to distinguish and diagnose small-bowel inflammatory or immune-related diseases, such as celiac disease.

1.3.2.7 Other Indications

Balloon-assisted enteroscopy can be utilized for shortening and straightening the bowel with overtube and balloons in cases wherein the normal anatomy has been altered by surgical resection. This technique can facilitate procedures such as endoscopic retrograde cholangiopancreatography and colonoscopy. In addition, it may be employed in percutaneous endoscopic jejunostomy placement for nutritional support.

1.3.3 Comparison Between Double- and Single-Balloon Enteroscopy

Previous studies comparing DBE and SBE have shown no significant differences in terms of diagnostic and therapeutic outcomes or complications even though there may be variations based on the operator's skill level and preference. Some reports have revealed that DBE has a higher total enteroscopy rate than SBE. However, this too can differ according to the endoscopist's expertise.

1.3.4 Contraindications

Balloon-assisted enteroscopy is relatively contraindicated in cases of severe small-bowel strictures with necrosis, strictures caused by previous abdominal surgeries, or fragile mucosa attributed to radiation or chemotherapy. The procedure duration is long, and it requires substantial skill. Hence, it should be cautiously considered in patients with severe respiratory or cardiovascular conditions and those who are hemodynamically unstable. The potential risks and benefits must be weighed before deciding to proceed or stop during the procedure. In addition, the transient elevation of amylase levels has been observed after oral insertion, which could exacerbate pancreatitis in susceptible patients. Thus, cautious decision-making is required.

1.3.5 Conclusion

The development of balloon-assisted enteroscopy has facilitated real-time assessment, biopsy-based diagnosis, and therapeutic intervention for small-bowel bleeding and obstructive lesions. This has expanded the understanding of clinicians regarding small-bowel diseases and prompted numerous related studies. By understanding the indications and contraindications and mastering the technique, small-bowel disorders can be effectively diagnosed and treated.

1.4 Clinical Outcomes of Balloon-Assisted Enteroscopy

1.4.1 Clinical Outcomes of Balloon-Assisted Enteroscopy

Double-balloon enteroscopy, introduced in 2001 and still in use today, has an overall diagnostic yield of 68% for small bowel diseases, according to a meta-analysis of nearly 10 years of research. Specific diagnostic rates include 68% for suspected small bowel bleeding, 63% for Crohn's disease, and 86% for small bowel obstruction. The most common findings from double-balloon enteroscopy were inflammatory lesions (33%), followed by vascular lesions (29%), tumors (23%), and diverticular diseases (4%). In cases of suspected small bowel bleeding, vascular lesions accounted for 40%, inflammatory lesions for 30%, tumors for 22%, and diverticular disease for 5%. The rate of complete small bowel examination (total enteroscopy) was 44%, and the incidence of serious complications, such as perforation, pancreatitis, bleeding, and aspiration pneumonia, was 0.72% [25].

Single-balloon enteroscopy offers advantages such as shorter preparation time and easier maneuverability compared to double-balloon enteroscopy. A meta-analysis of studies spanning 12 years found that single-balloon enteroscopy had an overall diagnostic yield of 62%, with 50% for suspected small bowel bleeding, 76% for Crohn's disease, 91% for tumorous lesions, 55% for unexplained abdominal pain, and 56% for unexplained diarrhea. In terms of enteroscopic findings, inflammatory lesions were the most common at 50%, followed by vascular lesions (26%), tumorous lesions (16%), and diverticular diseases (4%). The total enteroscopy rate was 22%, which increased slightly to 32% in studies after 2013. Serious complications occurred in 0.5% of cases [26].

1.4.1.1 Comparison of Efficacy and Safety Between Double-Balloon and Single-Balloon Enteroscopy

A meta-analysis comparing the efficacy of double-balloon and single-balloon enteroscopy found that the diagnostic yields for vascular lesions were 5–26% for single-balloon and 11–20% for double-balloon enteroscopy, while for tumorous lesions, the yields were 5–11% and 5–14%, respectively. There were no significant differences between the two methods regarding diagnostic yield, therapeutic yield, failure rates, or complete enteroscopy rates [27]. Korean studies reported no significant difference in the insertion depth between the two methods, but single-balloon enteroscopy had significantly shorter insertion and total procedure times compared to double-balloon enteroscopy in the antegrade approach. However, there were no statistically significant differences in diagnostic yield, therapeutic yield, or complication rates between the two methods [28].

1.4.1.2 Diagnostic and Therapeutic Outcomes of Balloon-Assisted Enteroscopy in Elderly Patients

The demand for small bowel enteroscopy in the elderly patients has been rising in recent years. A meta-analysis of balloon-assisted enteroscopy in patients aged 65 years and older found a diagnostic yield of 68% (68% for single-balloon and 67% for double-balloon enteroscopy) and a therapeutic yield of 45% (46% for single-balloon and 46% for double-balloon). The complication rate was reported at 2% for double-balloon enteroscopy only. A comparative meta-analysis of diagnostic yields in young and elderly patients showed that the diagnostic odds ratio was 1.83 for elderly patients (1.90 for single-balloon and 1.74 for double-balloon). The therapeutic yield odds ratio was 2.28, favoring elderly patients (2.36 for single-balloon and 2.20 for double-balloon), indicating better diagnostic and therapeutic outcomes in elderly patients. In terms of enteroscopy findings, Crohn's disease was most common in younger patients (37.1%), followed by angioectasia (16.3%) and tumors (14.7%), while angioectasia was most common in older patients (32.7%), followed by ulcers (13.4%) and tumors (12.7%). There were no significant differences in procedure-related complications between the younger and older groups [29].

1.4.2 Clinical Outcomes in Diagnosing Small Bowel Bleeding from Vascular Lesions

1.4.2.1 Clinical Outcomes of Balloon-Assisted Enteroscopy Versus Capsule Endoscopy

In diagnosing small bowel bleeding from vascular lesions, capsule endoscopy had a diagnostic rate of 59%, while double-balloon enteroscopy had a rate of 42%, indicating that capsule endoscopy performed better. Capsule endoscopy had a sensitivity of 93% and specificity of 82%. In contrast, double-balloon enteroscopy had a sensitivity of 84% and specificity of 92%, showing lower sensitivity but higher specificity than capsule endoscopy. The diagnostic yield for small bowel vascular lesions was 90% when capsule endoscopy was performed first, followed by balloon-assisted enteroscopy, compared to 83% when only balloon-assisted enteroscopy was used, reflecting a 7% improvement [30].

1.4.2.2 Clinical Outcomes of Balloon-Assisted Enteroscopy in Small Bowel Angioectasia Bleeding in Korea

In Korean multicenter study, data from 66 patients who underwent balloon-assisted enteroscopy for small bowel angioectasia bleeding were retrospectively reviewed. The study compared rebleeding rates between 45 patients who received endoscopic treatment and 21 patients who did not. The rebleeding rate was 15.6% in the treated group and 38.1% in the untreated group. Although the untreated group had a higher rebleeding rate, the difference was not statistically significant. Liver cirrhosis was identified as a risk factor for increased rebleeding risk, with a hazard ratio of 4.064 [31].

1.4.3 Clinical Outcomes of Balloon-Assisted Enteroscopy in Crohn's Disease Patients

1.4.3.1 Clinical Outcomes of Balloon Dilation for Crohn's Disease Strictures

A meta-analysis on the effectiveness of balloon-assisted enteroscopy for dilating small bowel strictures in Crohn's disease found a technical success rate of 95% and a short-term clinical efficacy of 82%. Graded dilation was positively correlated with clinical success, while new strictures, active disease in the jejunum/proximal ileum, and Asian ethnicity were negatively correlated. Major complications, including perforation, bleeding, and surgery related to dilation, occurred in about 5% of patients. During follow-up, 48% experienced recurrent obstructive symptoms, 39% required repeat dilation, and 27% underwent surgery. Active Crohn's disease in the jejunum or the proximal ileum increased the risk of reintervention, while patients on anti-tumor necrosis factor (TNF) agents had a lower risk of needing further procedures [32].

1.4.3.2 Clinical Outcomes of Balloon-Assisted Enteroscopy in Korean Patients with Crohn's Disease

A multicenter study by the Korean Association for the Study of Intestinal Diseases (KASID) retrospectively analyzed data from patients with Crohn's disease who underwent small bowel enteroscopy between 2004–2007 (early period) and 2008–2013 (late period). In both periods, the most common reason for enteroscopy was diagnosing Crohn's disease (50% in the early period vs. 31.1% in the late period, $p = 0.034$). However, procedures for investigating strictures and performing endoscopic treatments were more frequent in the late period (2.9% in the early period vs. 21.3% in the late period, $p = 0.002$). The diagnostic yield for suspected Crohn's disease was 90.7% in the early period and 95% in the late period. Therapeutic enteroscopy was commonly performed in the late period (5.1% in the early period vs. 17.6% in the late period, $p = 0.041$), with a procedural success rate of 100% in the early period and 80% in the late period. While the indications and diagnostic results for Crohn's disease remained unchanged, there was an increase in procedures for strictures and endoscopic treatments in the later period [33].

1.4.4 Conclusion

No significant differences were found in diagnostic yields, therapeutic yields, or complications between double-balloon and single-balloon enteroscopy. Performing capsule endoscopy prior to balloon-assisted enteroscopy enhances the diagnostic yield for small bowel lesions. Balloon-assisted enteroscopy is effective in diagnosing Crohn's disease, and its use in evaluating strictures and conducting therapeutic procedures, such as balloon dilation, is increasing. Although the technical success rate of balloon dilation is high, the potential risks of complications and recurrence should be carefully considered.

References

1. Yamamoto H. History and development of double balloon endoscopy. In: Mulder CJJ, editor. Atlas of double balloon endoscopy. 1st ed. Munich: Medconnect; 2007. p. 2.
2. Lewis BS. The history of enteroscopy. Gastrointest Endosc Clin N Am. 1999;9:1–11.
3. Tada M, Kawai K. Small bowel endoscopy. Scand J Gastroenterol. 1984;19:39–52.
4. Gostout CJ, Schroeder KW, Burton DD. Small bowel enteroscopy: an early experience in gastrointestinal bleeding of unknown origin. Gastrointest Endosc. 1991;37:5–8.
5. Shimizu S, Tada M, Kawai K. Development of a new insertion technique in push-type enteroscopy. Am J Gastro Enterol. 1987;82:844–7.
6. Appleyard M, Glukhovsky A, Swain P. Wireless-capsule diagnostic endoscopy for recurrent small-bowel bleeding. N Engl J Med. 2001;344:232–3.
7. Yamamoto H, Sekine Y, Sato Y, et al. Total enteroscopy with a nonsurgical steerable double-balloon method. Gastrointest Endosc. 2001;53:216–20.
8. Schneider M, Höllerich J, Beyna T. Device-assisted enteroscopy: a review of available techniques and upcoming new technologies. World J Gastroenterol. 2019;25:3538–45.
9. ASGE Technology Committee, Chauhan SS, Manfredi MA, et al. Enteroscopy. Gastrointest Endosc. 2015;82:975–90.
10. ASGE Technology Committee, DiSario JA, Petersen BT, et al. Enteroscopes. Gastrointest Endosc. 2007;66:872–80.
11. Yamamoto H, Despott EJ, González-Suárez B, Pennazio M, Mönkemüller K. The evolving role of device-assisted enteroscopy: the state of the art as of august 2023. Best Pract Res Clin Gastroenterol. 2023;64–65:101858.
12. Chauhan SS, Manfredi MA, Abu Dayyeh BK, et al. Enteroscopy. Gastrointest Endosc. 2015;82:975–90.
13. Hartmann D, Eickhoff A, Tamm R, Riemann JF. Balloon-assisted enteroscopy using a single-balloon technique. Endoscopy. 2007;39(Suppl 1):E276.
14. Neuhaus H, Beyna T, Schneider M, Devière J. Novel motorized spiral enteroscopy: first clinical case. VideoGIE. 2016;1:32–3.
15. Mussetto A, Merola E, Casadei C, et al. Device-assisted enteroscopy: are we ready to dismiss the spiral? World J Gastroenterol. 2024;30:3185–92.
16. Pennazio M. Enteroscopy in the diagnosis and management of obscure gastrointestinal bleeding. Gastrointest Endosc Clin N Am. 2009;19:409–26.
17. Abutalib H, Yano T, Shinozaki S, et al. Roles of capsule endoscopy and balloon-assisted enteroscopy in the optimal management of small bowel bleeding. Clin Endosc. 2020;53:402–9.
18. Yoo AY, Lee BJ, Kim WS, et al. Clinicopathologicalfeatures of small bowel tumors diagnosed by video capsule endoscopy and balloon-assisted enteroscopy: a single center experience. Clin Endosc. 2020;54:85–91.
19. Lee BI, Choi H, Choi KY, et al. Clinical characteristics of small bowel tumors diagnosed by double-balloon endoscopy: KASID multi-center study. Dig Dis Sci. 2011;56:2920–7.
20. Ohmiya N, Nakamura M, Takenaka H, et al. Management of small-bowel polyps in Peutz-Jeghers syndrome by using enteroclysis, double-balloon enteroscopy, and videocapsule endoscopy. Gastrointest Endosc. 2010;72:1209–16.

21. Kim J, Lee BJ, Ham NS, et al. Balloon-assisted enteroscopy for retrieval of small intestinal foreign bodies: a KASID multicenter study. Gastroenterol Res Pract. 2020;2020:3814267.
22. Domagk D, Mensink P, Aktas H, et al. Single- vs. double-balloon enteroscopy in small-bowel diagnostics: a randomized multicenter trial. Endoscopy. 2011;43:472–6.
23. Takano N, Yamada A, Watabe H, et al. Single-balloon versus double-balloon endoscopy for achieving total enteroscopy: a randomized, controlled trial. Gastrointest Endosc. 2011;73:734–9.
24. Kim TJ, Kim ER, Chang DK, et al. Comparison of theefficacy and safety of single-versus double-balloon enteroscopy performed by endoscopist experts in single-balloon enteroscopy: a single-center experience and meta-analysis. Gut Liver. 2017;11:520–7.
25. Xin L, Liao Z, Jiang YP, Li ZS. Indications, detectability, positive findings, total enteroscopy, and complications of diagnostic double-balloon endoscopy: a systematic review of data over the first decade of use. Gastrointest Endosc. 2011;74:563–70.
26. Gao Y, Xin L, Zhang YT, et al. Technical and clinical aspects of diagnostic single-balloon enteroscopy in the first decade of use: a systematic review and meta-analysis. Gut Liver. 2020;15:262–72.
27. Lipka S, Rabbanifard R, Kumar A, Brady P. Single versus double balloon enteroscopy for small bowel diagnostics: a systematic review and meta-analysis. J Clin Gastroenterol. 2015;49:177–84.
28. Kim TJ, Kim ER, Chang DK, Kim YH, Hong SN. Comparison of the efficacy and safety of single- versus double-balloon enteroscopy performed by endoscopist experts in single-balloon enteroscopy: a single-center experience and meta-analysis. Gut Liver. 2017;11:520–7.
29. Chetcuti Zammit S, Sanders DS, Sidhu R. Device assisted enteroscopy in the elderly – a systematic review and meta-analysis. Dig Liver Dis. 2019;51:1249–56.
30. Brito HP, Ribeiro IB, de Moura DTH, et al. Video capsule endoscopy vs double-balloon enteroscopy in the diagnosis of small bowel bleeding: a systematic review and meta-analysis. World J Gastrointest Endosc. 2018;10:400–21.
31. Jeon SR, Byeon JS, Jang HJ, et al. Clinical outcome after enteroscopy for small bowel angioectasia bleeding: a Korean Association for the Study of intestinal disease (KASID) multicenter study. J Gastroenterol Hepatol. 2017;32:388–94.
32. Bettenworth D, Bokemeyer A, Kou L, et al. Systematic review with meta-analysis: efficacy of balloon-assisted enteroscopy for dilation of small bowel Crohn's disease strictures. Aliment Pharmacol Ther. 2020;52:1104–16.
33. Jeon SR, Kim JO, Byeon JS, et al. Enteroscopy in Crohn's disease: are there any changes in role or outcomes over time? A KASID multicenter study. Gut Liver. 2021;15:375–82.

2 Double-Balloon Enteroscopy

Yehyun Park and Seong Ran Jeon

2.1 Introduction

The small bowel, measuring approximately 5–6 meters in length, is a tubular structure suspended within the abdominal cavity and anchored only by the mesentery. Its numerous complex loops and active peristalsis present challenges for comprehensive observation using conventional endoscopy, limiting the diagnosis and treatment of small bowel diseases. However, the development of double-balloon enteroscopy (DBE) in 2001 enabled complete visualization of the small bowel via transoral or transanal insertion. Utilizing air insufflation and washing, DBE allows for detailed lesion observation and facilitates tissue biopsy, manipulation, and therapeutic procedures, similar to standard enteroscopy, and overcomes the limitations of capsule endoscopy. This chapter provides an overview of DBE equipment, general and procedural preparations, and insertion techniques.

2.2 Equipment and Personnel

2.2.1 Enteroscope

Two DBE models, the EN-450 T5 and EN-450P5 (Fujinon Inc., Saitama, Japan), were introduced and remain in use. More recently, advanced models such as the therapeutic EN-580 T, the thinner EN-580XP, and the shorter 155 cm EI-580BT have been developed [1].

Y. Park
Ewha Womans University College of Medicine, Seoul, South Korea

S. R. Jeon (✉)
Soonchunhyang University College of Medicine, Seoul, South Korea
e-mail: 94jsr@hanmail.net

J.-J. Park et al. (eds.), *Balloon-Assisted Enteroscopy*,
https://doi.org/10.1007/978-981-95-2445-7_2

2.2.2 Fluoroscopy

The European Society of Gastrointestinal Endoscopy (ESGE) guidelines state that fluoroscopy is not mandatory but can be useful for achieving deep insertion of the enteroscope into the small bowel [1]. While experienced practitioners may achieve deep insertion without fluoroscopy, it can be an invaluable aid for beginners and even experienced practitioners when navigating small bowel loops and ensuring precise scope positioning.

2.2.3 Accessory Devices

DBE requires various accessory devices, including balloons attached to the enteroscope's tip, bands to secure the balloons, an overtube with its own balloon, and an air pump system for inflating and deflating the balloons. Attaching a transparent cap to the enteroscope tip is beneficial as it facilitates easier navigation of the intestinal lumen with minimal air insufflation. This approach, commonly used in colonoscopy, helps prevent overdistension and is especially advantageous during therapeutic procedures such as hemostasis or polypectomy, except in cases where strictures are suspected.

2.2.4 Personnel

A typical DBE procedure requires at least four personnel, including the primary operator. Two assistants are typically required. One to manage the air pump system or secure the overtube and the other to monitor the patient, administer medications, and assist with tasks such as biopsies or clipping. The team generally consists of one medical technician, two nurses, and one physician. In some settings, an additional physician may be included to manage sedation, resulting in a five-member team.

2.2.5 CO_2 Insufflator

Continuous gas insufflation into the small bowel can make it difficult to shorten the bowel and achieve adequate insertion. Carbon dioxide (CO_2) gas, which is 100 times more soluble in water than air, is rapidly absorbed and expelled through respiration. CO_2 insufflation improves insertion depth and enhances the likelihood of visualizing the entire small bowel [2]. Additionally, it reduces patient discomfort and pain associated with bowel distension during and after lengthy procedures, typically those exceeding 1 h. The ESGE recommends CO_2 for small bowel enteroscopy [1].

2.3 General Preparations

Preparation for DBE depends on the chosen insertion route, which is determined by the patient's symptoms (e.g., hematochezia, melena) and prior diagnostic results (e.g., upper gastrointestinal endoscopy, colonoscopy, capsule endoscopy, or small bowel imaging with computed tomography [CT] or magnetic resonance imaging [MRI]). If the objective is to examine the entire small bowel, the procedure is divided into two sessions: one for transoral insertion and another for transanal insertion. Conversely, if the focus is on a specific lesion identified in previous tests, the route providing the closest access to the lesion is selected first.

2.3.1 Consent Form

Before conducting DBE, obtain informed consent with particular attention to the patient's surgical history. Prior surgeries can result in adhesions or altered anatomy, complicating DBE insertion or requiring additional caution. Review the surgical history in detail, including anastomosis methods. Confirm the patient's personal details, current medications, underlying conditions, bleeding risks, airway anomalies, and the potential presence of intestinal strictures or obstructions. Clearly explain the examination's necessity, purpose, process, benefits, limitations, and potential complications. While complications are uncommon, they can occur even in diagnostic procedures due to the procedure's duration and the use of deep sedation or general anesthesia. Reported complication rates are approximately 0.8% for diagnostic procedures and up to 8% for therapeutic procedures. Major complications include perforation, bleeding, acute pancreatitis, and sedation-related issues. Ensure these risks, alternative diagnostic options, the prognosis without the examination, and the possibility of procedural modifications or extensions are fully explained and documented in the consent form.

2.3.2 Fasting and Bowel Preparation

As with other endoscopic procedures, the effectiveness of bowel preparation and the presence of residual matter significantly influence the detection of lesions during DBE. Residual food or fecal matter can increase friction between the enteroscope and the overtube, making the procedure more challenging.

2.3.3 Transoral Examination

For transoral insertion, fasting is typically sufficient. Solid food should be avoided for 8–12 h and liquids for 4–6 h before the procedure [1]. However, in cases of slow gastrointestinal motility, suspected strictures, ongoing oral iron supplementation, or prior abdominal surgeries where residual matter is anticipated, or deep insertion is required, a bowel preparation solution is recommended [1, 3].

2.3.4 Transanal Examination

For transanal insertion, inadequate bowel preparation can hinder enteroscope insertion, requiring preparation similar to that for colonoscopy. Patients should follow a low-residue or prescribed diet the day before the procedure, and a split-dose bowel preparation is recommended for the best results.

2.3.5 Sedation

Sedation is required for DBE due to its prolonged duration and the discomfort caused by air insufflation and repeated insertion and withdrawal of the enteroscope and overtube [1, 3]. Moderate sedation, deep sedation, and general anesthesia can be used. Transoral insertion typically requires deep sedation because of frequent belching, nausea, vomiting, and abdominal pain, while moderate sedation is usually adequate for transanal insertion [4]. Although research on the effect of specific sedatives on DBE success or insertion depth is limited, common practice includes using benzodiazepines like midazolam and analgesics like pethidine for standard sedation during transanal insertion, with propofol added for deeper sedation during transoral insertion. Studies comparing endoscopist-directed nurse-administered sedation with monitored anesthesia care (MAC) by an anesthesiologist have shown no significant differences in outcomes or complications, making endoscopist-directed sedation a safe option [5]. However, sedation levels and methods should be adjusted according to patient factors, including underlying conditions, overall health, expected procedure duration, and need for therapeutic intervention. For high-risk patients or when deep sedation is required, MAC with an anesthesiologist may be recommended [4].

The preparations and sedation methods for DBE based on the insertion route are summarized in Table 2.1.

Table 2.1 Preparation and sedation methods for DBE based on the insertion route

	Preparation	Sedation
Transoral examination	Fasting is typically sufficient Solid food: 8–12 h Liquid food: 4–6 h	Moderate or deep sedation
Transanal examination	Bowel preparation similar to colonoscopy required	Moderate sedation

2.4 Procedure Preparation

2.4.1 Instruments

The DBE system includes a specialized enteroscope with a balloon at its distal end, an overtube with its own balloon, and a balloon controller to manage inflation or deflation. The balloon controller regulates and monitors the inflation pressure of both the enteroscope and overtube balloons. The pressure is set to 45 mm Hg, which is the minimum necessary to hold the small bowel for enteroscope insertion while minimizing abdominal pain or discomfort from balloon inflation. If the overtube is inserted beyond the 155-cm mark on the enteroscope shaft, indicated by the white line, it may damage the balloon on the enteroscope. This point marks the maximum insertion depth for the overtube (Fig. 2.1).

2.4.2 Insufflation

Air insufflation during DBE can cause overdistension of the small bowel, which may hinder bowel shortening and lead to abdominal pain. A meta-analysis showed that the visual analog scale at 6 h favored CO_2 over room air. CO_2 also improved transoral insertion depth and total enteroscopy rates, and the mean dose of propofol was lower in the CO_2 group compared to air. However, there were no significant differences in adverse events between the two groups [5].

2.5 Insertion Technique

2.5.1 Principle of DBE [7]

DBE employs a push-and-pull method, where the enteroscope and overtube are alternately inflated and deflated in a cycle of forward movement and withdrawal. This process continues until the maximum insertion point or target lesion is reached (Fig. 2.2). Simply inserting the enteroscope into the small bowel can cause bending and form a large loop, making further insertion difficult due to poor transmission of force to the enteroscope tip. However, using the balloon on the overtube tip as a fixation point prevents excessive stretching of the small bowel, making it easier to

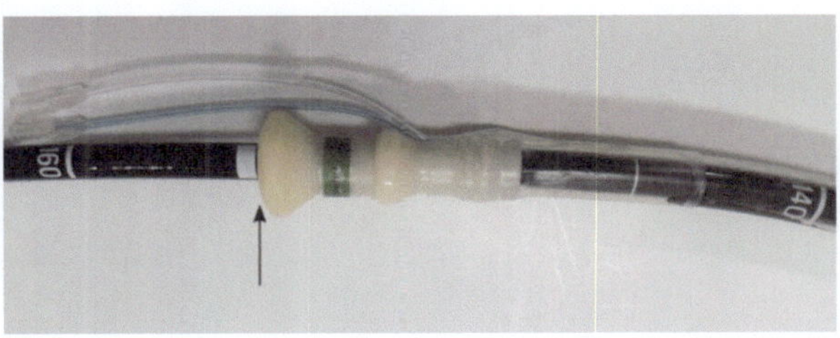

Fig. 2.1 Maximum insertion depth (indicated by the white line as a distance marker at 155 cm on the enteroscope shaft) of the overtube

advance the enteroscope. After deflating the overtube balloon and inflating the enteroscope balloon, the overtube is inserted along the enteroscope until it reaches the tip ("push" procedure). Both the enteroscope and the overtube are then pulled back with the balloons inflated to secure the small bowel ("pull" procedure). Once the overtube balloon is inflated to hold the small bowel, the enteroscope balloon is deflated to allow the enteroscope to advance into the deeper small bowel. This cycle is repeated, gradually allowing the enteroscope to move further from the overtube balloon, which serves as the fixation point.

2.5.2 Transoral Insertion [7, 8]

DBE is typically performed by two people: an endoscopist and an assistant who controls the overtube (Fig. 2.3). The steps for transoral insertion are as follows (Fig. 2.4). For deep insertion, it is recommended that the enteroscope forms a counterclockwise concentric circle (Fig. 2.5a):

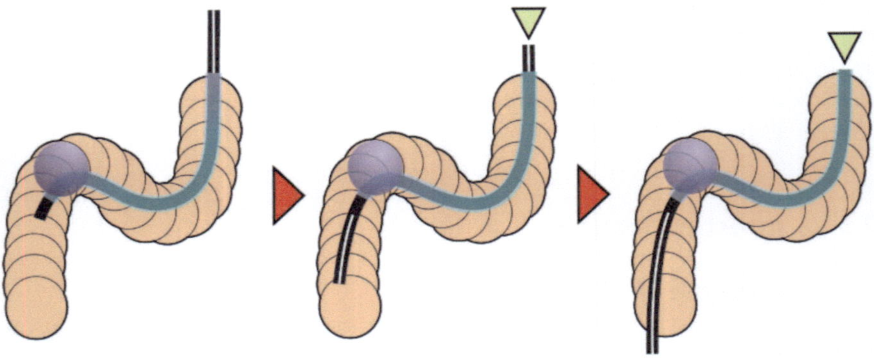

Fig. 2.2 Principle of double-balloon enteroscopy

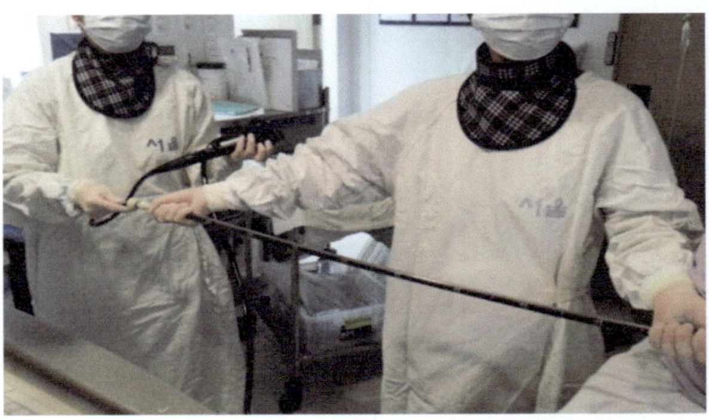

Fig. 2.3 Double-balloon enteroscopy: a two-person procedure

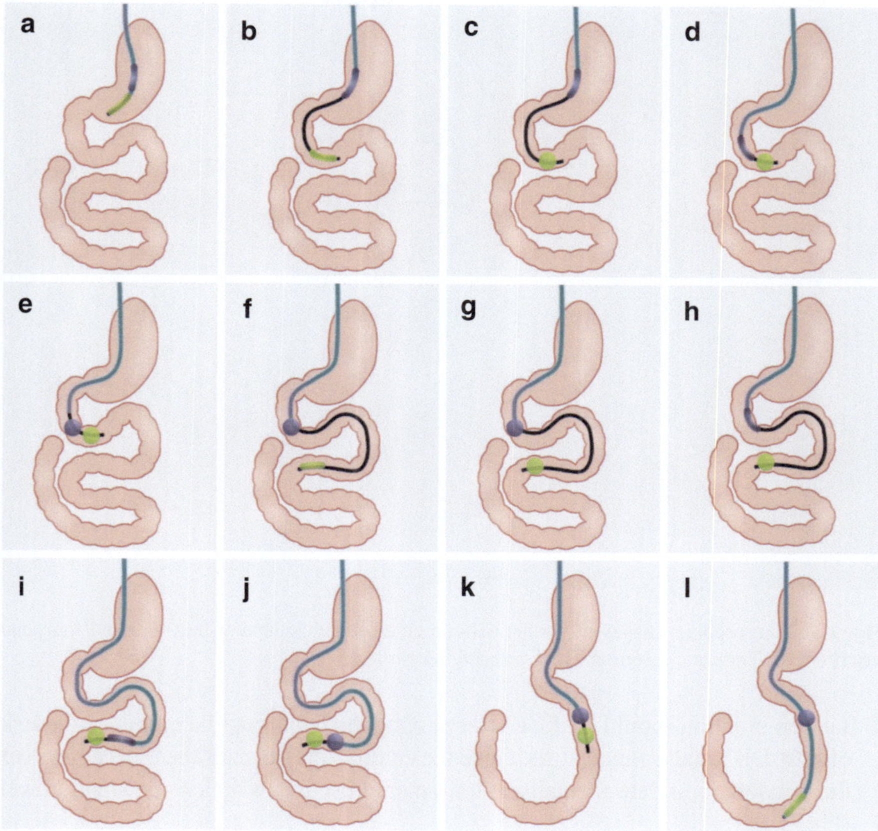

Fig. 2.4 Step-by-step process of transoral insertion in double-balloon enteroscopy. (**a**) Insert the enteroscope through the overtube into the stomach. (**b** and **c**) Advance the enteroscope as far as possible into the third portion of the duodenum and inflate the balloon on the enteroscope to secure the small bowel. (**d** and **e**) Move the overtube along the enteroscope to the third portion of the duodenum and inflate the balloon on the overtube to grip the small bowel. (**f–i**) Deflate the balloon on the enteroscope and advance it as far as possible into the proximal jejunum. (**j** and **k**) With both balloons inflated, gently withdraw the enteroscope and overtube together to shorten the jejunum. (**l**) Inflate the balloon on the overtube to grip the small bowel and advance the enteroscope to the deep small bowel

① As with esophagogastroduodenoscopy, after the overtube is attached to the enteroscope, one operator inserts only the enteroscope until it reaches the stomach. Then, the assistant inserts the overtube along the enteroscope (Fig. 2.4a). Care should be taken to avoid inserting the overtube beyond the white line, which serves as a distance marker at 155 cm on the enteroscope shaft. The assistant then holds the overtube firmly in a straight line while the operator advances it to the second part of the duodenum.

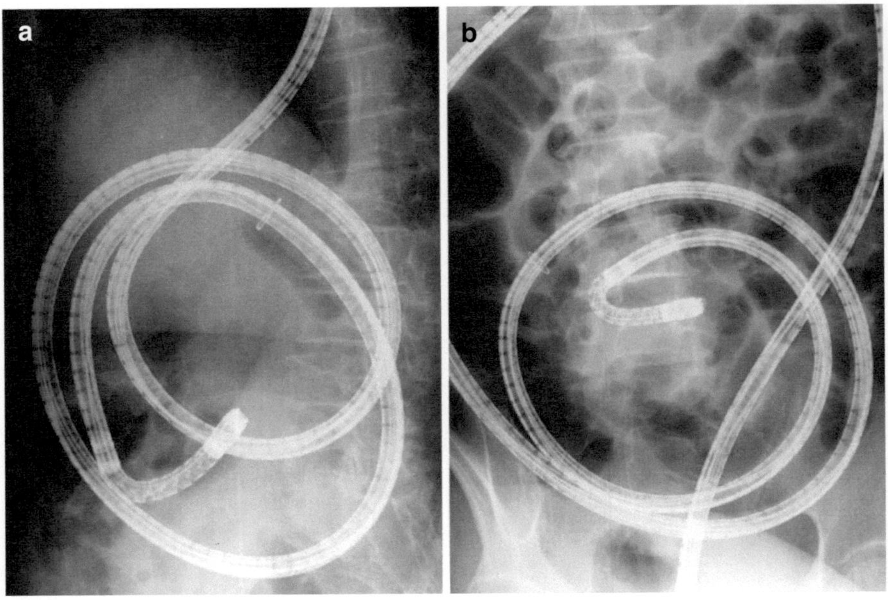

Fig. 2.5 Fluoroscopic images of double-balloon enteroscopy following transoral and transanal insertion. (**a**) Transoral insertion. (**b**) Transanal insertion

② Balloon inflation should be done after passing the major papilla to reduce the risk of post-DBE acute pancreatitis. Once the enteroscope reaches the third portion of the duodenum, inflate the balloon on the enteroscope to secure the small bowel (Fig. 2.4b, c).

③ Advance the overtube to the third portion of the duodenum along the enteroscope, and inflate the balloon on the overtube to grip the jejunum (Fig. 2.4d, e).

④ Deflate the balloon on the enteroscope and advance it as far as possible into the proximal jejunum (Fig. 2.5f–i). Then, retract both the enteroscope and overtube while keeping both balloons inflated to shorten the jejunum (Fig. 2.4j, k).

⑤ Inflate only the balloon on the overtube to grip the small bowel, then deflate the balloon on the enteroscope to continue advancing it into the deep small bowel (Fig. 2.4l).

2.5.3 Transanal Insertion [7, 8]

Since the enteroscope must pass through the colon to reach the small bowel, transanal insertion can be more difficult than transoral insertion. The enteroscope and the overtube are advanced to the cecum, either directly or using the previously mentioned push–pull technique. Transanal DBE can be challenging in cases of a long, looped colon, a large cecum, retroflexed ileocecal valve, or fixed terminal ileum. The procedure is generally performed similarly to transoral insertion, with the insertion made by creating a counterclockwise circular loop, like in the colon (Fig. 2.5b):

① One operator inserts the enteroscope about 45 cm (sigmoid colon) from the anus, similar to colonoscopy, without the overtube.
② Inflate only the balloon on the enteroscope to secure the colon, and then the assistant inserts the overtube along the enteroscope.
③ Inflate the balloons on both the enteroscope and overtube to secure the sigmoid colon, and then pull both the enteroscope and overtube back with the balloons inflated to shorten the sigmoid colon. Deflate the balloon on the enteroscope to proceed toward the descending colon. If there is adhesion in the sigmoid colon, the enteroscope is inserted into the proximal portion first, without following the previous step. The overtube helps prevent bending and stretching of loops without fully straightening the sigmoid colon.
④ Upon reaching the splenic flexure, inflate the balloon on the enteroscope to secure the colon. Position the overtube at the splenic flexure and inflate the balloon on the overtube.
⑤ After securing the splenic flexure with the overtube balloon, deflate the balloon on the enteroscope to advance toward the transverse colon. In some cases, the cecum can be reached with enteroscope manipulation alone. However, in cases with ptosis of the midtransverse colon or an angulated hepatic flexure, the procedure may be difficult. By positioning the enteroscope and overtube at the hepatic flexure and inflating both balloons to shorten the colon, the hepatic flexure can become obtuse. Inflating the overtube balloon to secure the colon allows the enteroscope to be more easily advanced to the cecum (Fig. 2.6).
⑥ Once the colon is sufficiently shortened, the enteroscope can be easily passed through the ileocecal valve. Position the valve at 9 o'clock and advance directly through it. In some cases, the enteroscope may struggle to pass over the ileocecal valve. To facilitate this, the overtube is inserted into the ascending colon, and both balloons are inflated to secure the colon. One method involves inserting the enteroscope after pulling back the ascending colon to create a wider angle between the ascending colon and terminal ileum.

Another method involves pushing the enteroscope after it is turned in the cecum. Applying abdominal pressure can also assist in advancing the enteroscope into the terminal ileum when retroflexion occurs in the cecum.

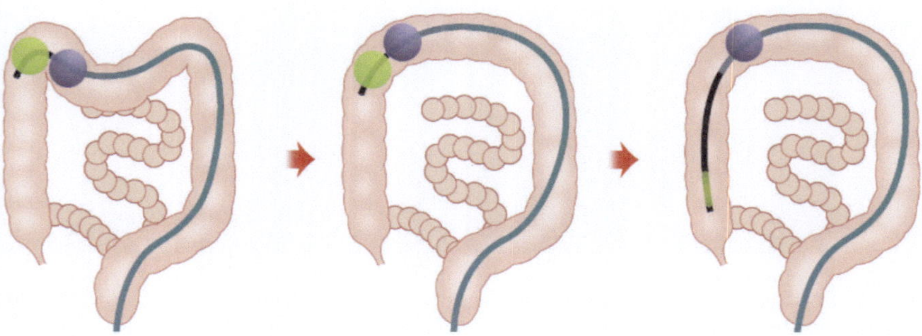

Fig. 2.6 Approach for challenging ileocecal valve insertion

⑦ When trying to shorten the terminal ileum to pass over the ileocecal valve, the enteroscope may slip into the cecum. After passing through the ileocecal valve, both the enteroscope and the overtube are advanced as far as possible, and the first attempt at shortening is made. The balloon on the enteroscope is inflated to secure the ileum, and then the overtube balloon is deflated to allow the overtube to reach the white line. The balloon on the overtube is inflated to grip the ileum, and then the enteroscope balloon is deflated to move the enteroscope further into the ileum, continuing in a manner similar to transoral insertion process.

2.5.4 Tips for Deep Insertion of the Enteroscope

① To advance the enteroscope further, it should be inserted while forming a small bowel loop in a counterclockwise direction. In transoral insertion with clockwise rotation, a large intragastric loop often forms when the operator pushes the scope to advance it, making deep insertion difficult without unwanted looping (Fig. 2.7). In transanal insertion with clockwise rotation, the enteroscope may become fixed within the pelvis. Therefore, if a clockwise circle is formed or a concentric circle cannot be created, rotate the enteroscope and overtube counterclockwise under fluoroscopy guidance to create a counterclockwise concentric circle [4].

② Avoid inserting the enteroscope when it is severely bent by lifting the distal end or bending it too far to the left or right. In such cases, it is important to return the enteroscope to a neutral position as much as possible to reduce the force on the distal end before attempting the next insertion.

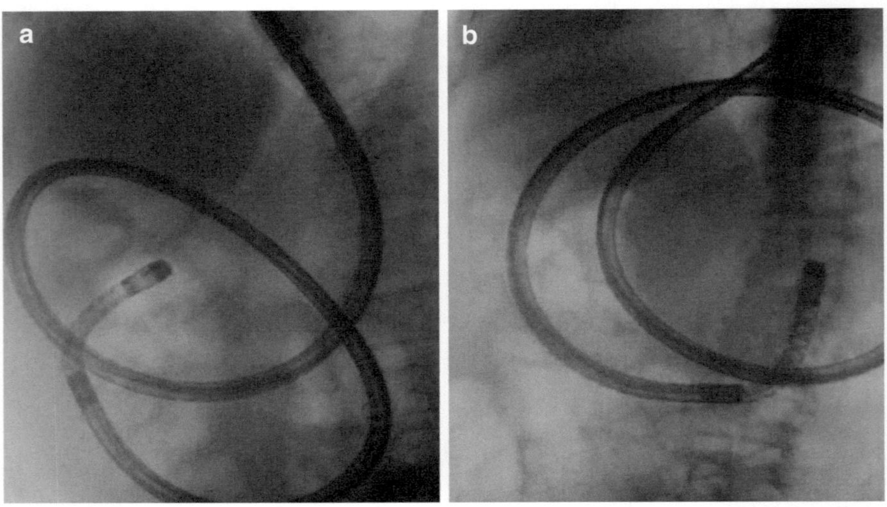

Fig. 2.7 Small bowel loop during transoral insertion of double-balloon enteroscopy. (**a**) Clockwise direction with large intragastric loop. (**b**) Counterclockwise direction without redundant loop

③ When a sharp angle or complex loop forms in the small bowel, the force applied to the enteroscope shaft may not effectively reach the tip. Fluoroscopy can help determine how to straighten the proximal end and when to stop shortening.

References

1. Rondonotti E, Spada C, Adler S, May A, Despott EJ, Koulaouzidis A, et al. Small-bowel capsule endoscopy and device-assisted enteroscopy for diagnosis and treatment of small-bowel disorders: European Society of Gastrointestinal Endoscopy (ESGE) technical review. Endoscopy. 2018;50:423–46.
2. Lenz P, Meister T, Manno M, Pennazio M, Conigliaro R, Lebkucher S, et al. CO2 insufflation during single-balloon enteroscopy: a multicenter randomized controlled trial. Endoscopy. 2014;46:53–8.
3. May A. Double-balloon enteroscopy. Gastrointest Endosc Clin N Am. 2017;27:113–22.
4. Kim J. Training in endoscopy: enteroscopy. Clin Endosc. 2017;50:328–33.
5. Judah JR, Collins D, Gaidos JK, Hou W, Forsmark CE, Draganov PV. Prospective evaluation of gastroenterologist-guided, nurse-administered standard sedation for spiral deep small bowel enteroscopy. Dig Dis Sci. 2010;55:2584–91.
6. Shiani A, Lipka S, Lai A, Rodriquez AC, Andrade CM, Kumar A, et al. Carbon dioxide versus room air insufflation during balloon-assisted enteroscopy: a systematic review with meta-analysis. Endosc Int Open. 2017;5:E67–75.
7. Sunada K, Yamamoto H. Double balloon enteroscopy: techniques. Ther Adv Gastroenterol. 2008;10:46–53.
8. Yang DH. Insertion techniques of enteroscopy: in normal and altered anatomy. In 49th seminar of Korean Society of Gastrointestinal Endoscopy; 2013

3 Single-Balloon Enteroscopy

Jinsu Kim

3.1 Introduction

The single-balloon enteroscope, introduced by Olympus (Tokyo, Japan) in 2006 and commercially available since 2007, differs significantly from the double-balloon enteroscope (DBE) developed by Fujinon (now Fujifilm, Tokyo, Japan). The primary distinction is that the single-balloon enteroscopy (SBE) lacks a balloon at the tip of the endoscope, a feature present in the DBE. Another key difference lies in the materials used: while Fujinon initially employed latex balloons and a polyurethane overtube, Olympus uses silicone-based overtubes and balloons, making SBE a better option for patients with latex allergies. Fujifilm has since updated its products to include non-latex overtubes.

The SBE is slightly more rigid than the DBE, which improves maneuverability during procedures. Its air-infusion pump is also simpler, enabling inflation and deflation of the overtube balloon with a single button, thereby reducing preparation time. However, the absence of a tip balloon in the SBE requires the enteroscope tip to be bent and hooked into the small bowel to prevent it from slipping backward while manipulating the overtube.

A notable drawback of the SBE is its lower total enteroscopy rate compared to the DBE (0–25% vs. 40–80%). However, clinical studies indicate that despite this limitation, both methods offer similar diagnostic and therapeutic yields for small bowel diseases [1]. The performance of the SBE can be enhanced by using a CO_2 insufflator and attaching a transparent cap to the endoscope tip [2], which may increase the total enteroscopy rate to match that of the DBE.

J. Kim (✉)
College of Medicine, The Catholic University of Korea, Seoul, South Korea
e-mail: jinsu23@naver.com

J.-J. Park et al. (eds.), *Balloon-Assisted Enteroscopy*,
https://doi.org/10.1007/978-981-95-2445-7_3

3.2 Components of the Single-Balloon Enteroscopy (SBE)

3.2.1 Enteroscope (SIF-Q180)

The total length of the SBE was 2345 mm, with a working length of 2000 mm (Fig. 3.1). The distal tip of insertion tube have a diameter of 9.2 mm. It offers a 140° field of view with angulation ranges of 180° up and down and 160° left and right. The 2.8-mm working channel accommodates standard instruments such as biopsy forceps, injection needles, and resection snares. However, this channel has limitations in deploying conventional through-the-scope metallic stents [3].

3.2.2 Overtube (Splint Tube, ST-SB1)

The Olympus overtube (ST-SB1) has an outer diameter of 13.2 mm and an inner diameter of 11 mm. Its total length is 1400 mm, with a working length of 1320 mm (Fig. 3.2). Made of silicone, the overtube and its distal-end balloon feature a hydrophilic lubricant coating on the inner surface. This coating minimizes friction during the insertion and withdrawal of the endoscope.

3.2.3 Air Infusion Pump (Olympus Balloon Control Unit, OBCU)

This device is designed to inflate and deflate the overtube balloon, with the current balloon pressure displayed numerically (Fig. 3.3). The standard air pressure is set at 5.4 kPa, and an alarm is triggered if the pressure exceeds 8.2 kPa, prompting a necessary deflation to reduce the pressure.

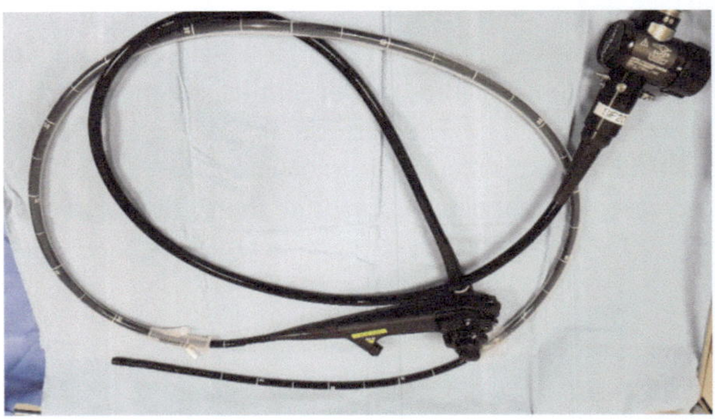

Fig. 3.1 Single-balloon enteroscope (SIF-Q180, Olympus, Tokyo, Japan)

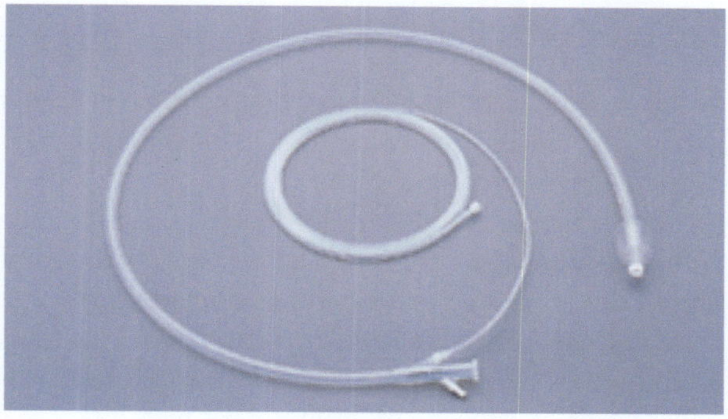

Fig. 3.2 Olympus overtube (ST-SB1)

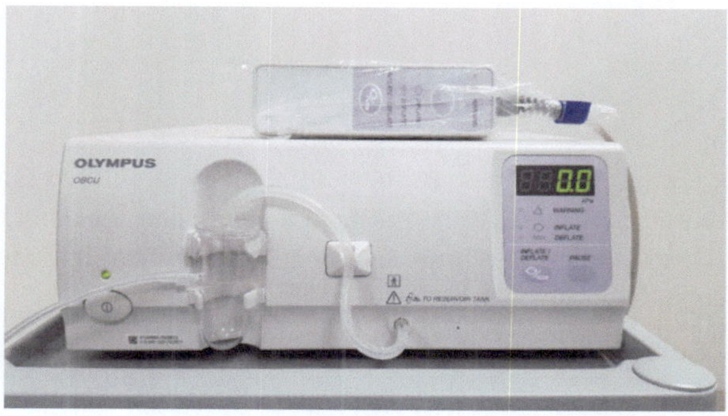

Fig. 3.3 Olympus balloon control unit

3.3 Preparations Before the Enteroscope Procedure

3.3.1 Antegrade Enteroscopy

This approach is primarily used for examining the jejunum. Patients are typically required to fast for around 8 h before the procedure, following a preparation process similar to that of an upper gastrointestinal endoscopy.

3.3.2 Retrograde Enteroscopy

This method is mainly performed to observe the ileum. The bowel preparation process is the same as that used for a colonoscopy.

3.3.3 Sedation Method

While general anesthesia in an operating room is used in some countries, the procedure in Korea is usually performed under conscious sedation, similar to other sedated endoscopic procedures.

Commonly used sedatives for the procedure include **midazolam** and **propofol,** with **pethidine** often given to manage pain and discomfort. Due to the longer duration of the procedure compared to standard upper or lower gastrointestinal endoscopy and the larger diameter of the overtube, patients may experience increased discomfort. If the procedure is prolonged and the effects of sedation diminish, additional doses of midazolam, propofol, or pethidine can be administered to maintain adequate sedation.

3.4 Patient Monitoring

Patients' vital signs must be continuously monitored throughout the procedure. The monitoring protocol is the same as that used for other endoscopic procedures performed under conscious sedation, ensuring patient safety and prompt detection of any adverse events.

3.5 Preparation of the Overtube

3.5.1 Saline Infusion Inside the Overtube (Fig. 3.4)

3.5.2 Balloon Test (Figs. 3.5 and 3.6)

3.5.3 Connection of the Enteroscope and Overtube

After attaching the enteroscope to the overtube, test its movement by sliding the enteroscope back and forth to ensure smooth motion without resistance (Fig. 3.7). If resistance occurs, inject additional saline into the overtube or check for any foreign material on the surface of the enteroscope or inside the overtube.

3.5.4 Attachment of a Transparent Cap to the Distal End

Attach a transparent cap to the distal end of the enteroscope (Fig. 3.8). This cap has an outer diameter of 11 mm and extends approximately 4 mm beyond the end of the scope. Although the procedure can be performed without the cap, its use generally

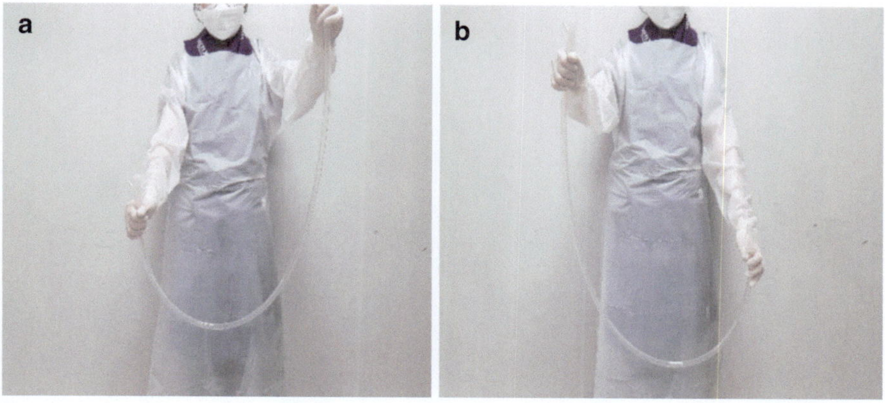

Fig. 3.4 Overtube preparation. To prepare ~ prepare the overtube, inject 50 cc of saline into it and gently shake it from side to side. This activates the hydrophilic lubricant coating on the inner surface of the overtube, enhancing its lubricating properties

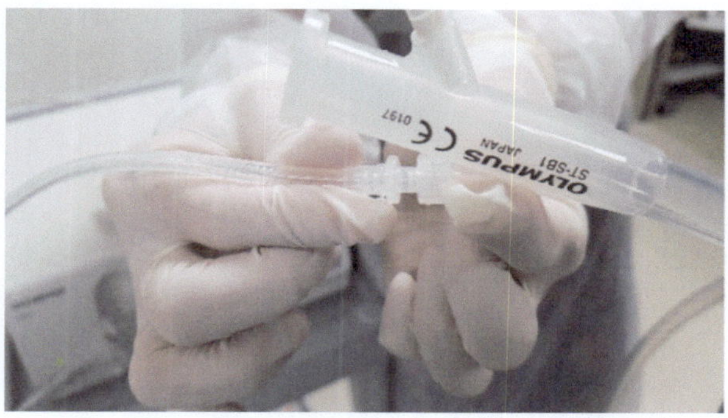

Fig. 3.5 The connection between the the air infusion tube of the Olympus Balloon Control Unit (OBCU) and the air inlet port of the overtube

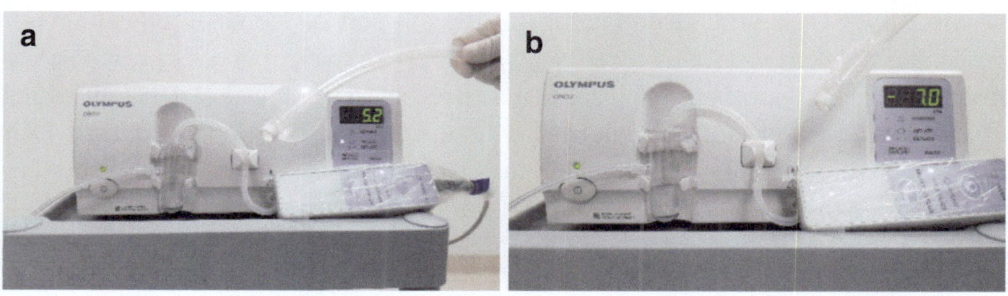

Fig. 3.6 Balloon inflation check. To ensure ~ ensure proper function, press the air infusion button on the OBCU to inflate the balloon, checking for proper inflation and an increase in pressure. Then, press the button again to deflate the balloon, verifying that the pressure gauge shows a negative reading

facilitates smoother insertion and enhances stability during the procedure. However, if prior radiologic imaging or endoscopic findings suggest the presence of a small bowel stricture and access beyond the stricture is required, the cap may impede

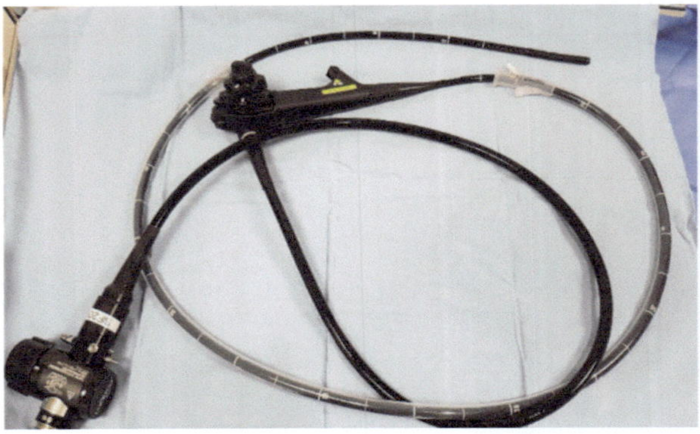

Fig. 3.7 Small bowel enteroscope combined with the overtube

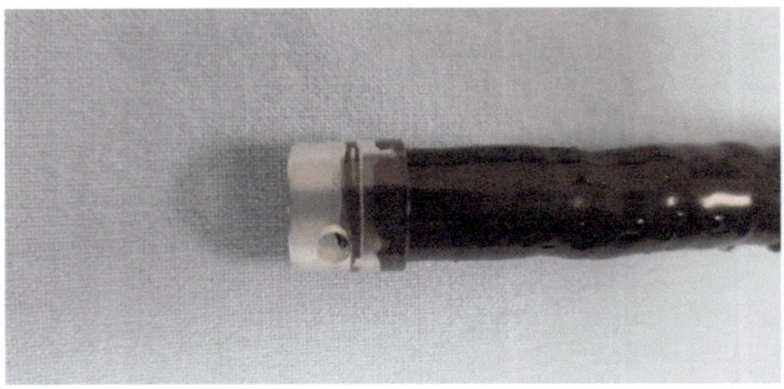

Fig. 3.8 Olympus distal attachment (D-201-10704)

scope passage. In such cases, removing the cap before the procedure is recommended.

3.5.5 Testing the Co_2 Insufflator

Connect the CO_2 insufflator to the air insufflation port of the small bowel enteroscope and confirm proper CO_2 delivery (Fig. 3.9). While room air can be used to maintain a clear endoscopic field, it may cause excessive bowel distension, which can hinder the bowel shortening necessary for deep scope insertion. In contrast, CO_2 is absorbed more rapidly than room air, making it more effective for bowel shortening. Additionally, CO_2 reduces abdominal discomfort associated with excessive air insufflation [2, 4].

3.5.6 Use of Fluoroscopy Equipment

Fluoroscopy is utilized during small bowel enteroscopy to monitor the formation of the circular loop required for deep bowel insertion (Fig. 3.10a). If a reverse loop is identified, it must be corrected to a proper circular loop to facilitate further advancement of the enteroscope (Fig. 3.10b). Fluoroscopy is particularly helpful for reaching the deep small bowel. However, if the lesion is suspected to be in the proximal

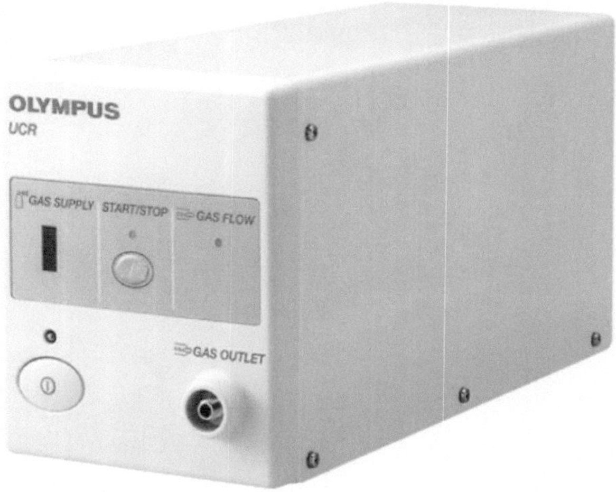

Fig. 3.9 Olympus CO_2 regulation unit (UCR)

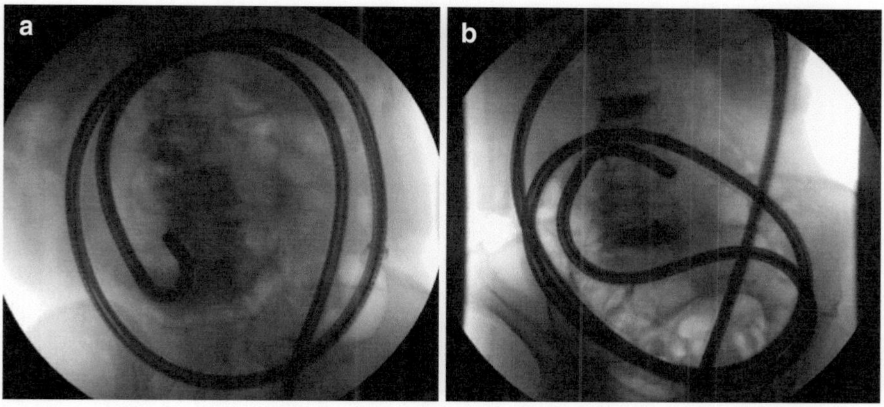

Fig. 3.10 (**a**) Circular loop. To advance into the deep small bowel, the pushing force applied to the small bowel enteroscope is effectively transmitted to the distal end. (**b**) Reverse loop. When a reverse loop occurs, the pushing force applied to the small bowel enteroscope is not effectively transmitted to the distal end due to the dispersion of force caused by the loop

jejunum or the distal ileum, where deep insertion is unnecessary, the procedure can be performed in a standard endoscopy room without fluoroscopy. As practitioners gain more experience with small bowel enteroscopy, the reliance on fluoroscopy tends to decrease [5].

3.6 Insertion Method

3.6.1 General Insertion Technique for SBE (Fig. 3.11)

After inserting the endoscope, adjust the distal tip upward or downward to hook onto the intestinal mucosa, securing the tip in place. Then, deflate the balloon and

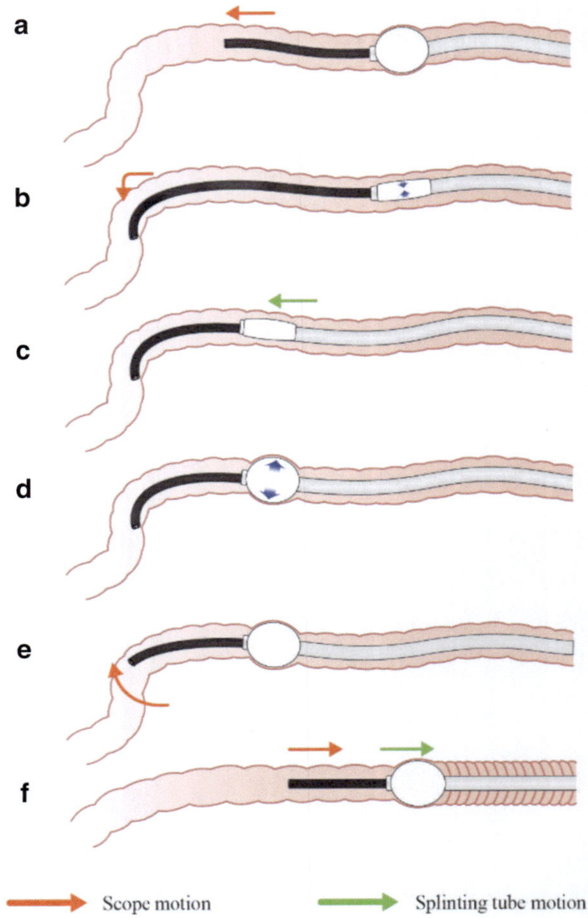

Fig. 3.11 Insertion method of the SBE

advance the overtube. Once the overtube is in position, reinflate the balloon to fix the overtube to the intestinal lumen. Next, return the distal tip to the neutral position and pull both the endoscope and overtube simultaneously to shorten the bowel. After shortening, reinsert the endoscope and repeat the process.

① Insert the scope as deeply as possible. ② Angulate the scope to secure the intestinal tract and deflate the balloon. ③ Advance the splinting tube. ④ Inflate the balloon. ⑤ Release the angulation. ⑥ Withdraw the splinting tube and scope to shorten the intestinal tract.

3.6.2 Antegrade Insertion (Fig. 3.12)

For antegrade insertion, patients are positioned in a manner similar to endoscopic retrograde cholangiopancreatography (prone position). The assistant holds the

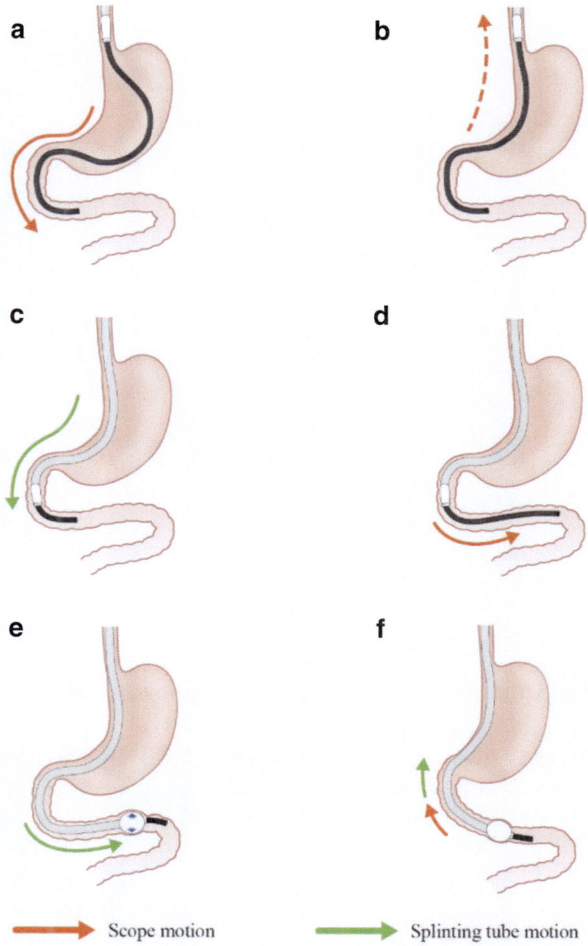

Fig. 3.12 Antegrade insertion. ① Bend the scope when inserting it from the stomach into the duodenum. ② Stretch the scope by pulling back the enteroscope. ③ Advance the splinting tube until it passes the pyloric ring. ④ Continue to insert the scope further. ⑤ Advance the overtube to the tip of the enteroscope, and inflate the overtube balloon to anchor it securely to the small bowel. ⑥ Withdraw the splinting tube and the scope to shorten the intestinal tract

enteroscope and overtube, while the endoscopist controls the enteroscope. This technique is referred to as the "two-man method" (Fig. 3.13).

Recently, the "single-man method" has been introduced, where the endoscopist operates both the overtube and the enteroscope independently, without an assistant (Fig. 3.14). In this method, the endoscopist must handle the overtube and the endoscope simultaneously, using some fingers to pull the overtube while the remaining fingers and palm are used to insert the endoscope. This technique is known as the "grip and pinch technique." [6]

3.6.3 Retrograde Insertion (Fig. 3.15)

The general technique for retrograde insertion is similar to that of a standard colonoscopy. However, since the enteroscope is more flexible than a typical

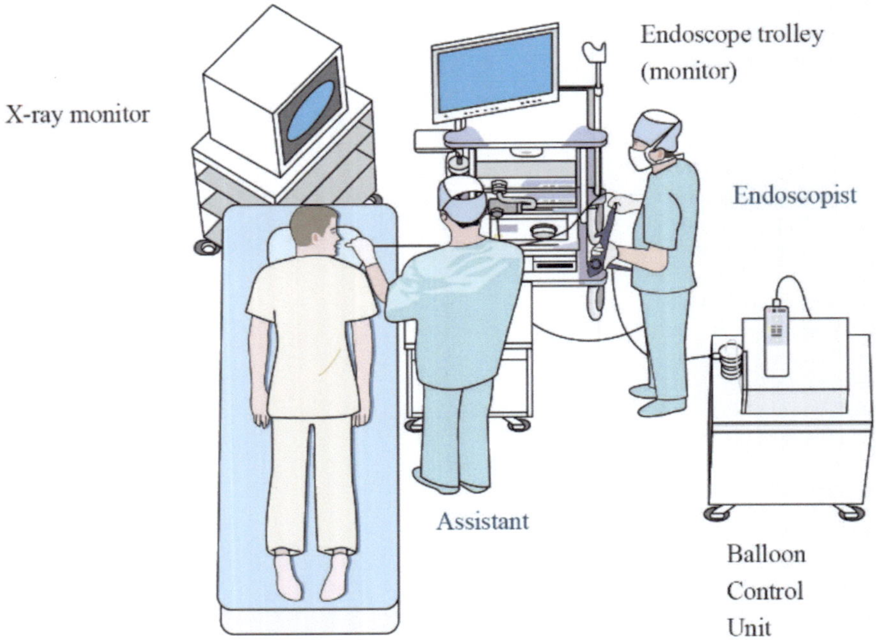

Fig. 3.13 Example of antegrade insertion (two-man method)

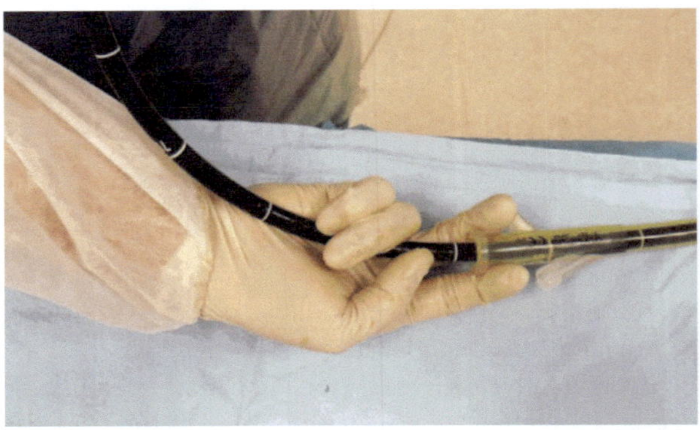

Fig. 3.14 Grip and pinch technique. The operator grips the enteroscope behind the overtube, between the third and fifth fingers, with the palm while pinching the overtube with the first and second fingers

colonoscope, it can be more easily advanced to the descending colon. Once the enteroscope reaches the descending colon, the overtube is advanced near the tip of the enteroscope. After inflating the overtube balloon to secure it in place, gently pull back to straighten the colon. Then, deflate the balloon, reinsert the enteroscope, and advance the overtube again. This process is repeated to progress to the ascending colon.

After advancing the enteroscope to the ascending colon, the bowel must be shortened to reduce the angle for entry into the terminal ileum. If the angle is not sufficiently reduced, looping may occur when attempting to insert the enteroscope into

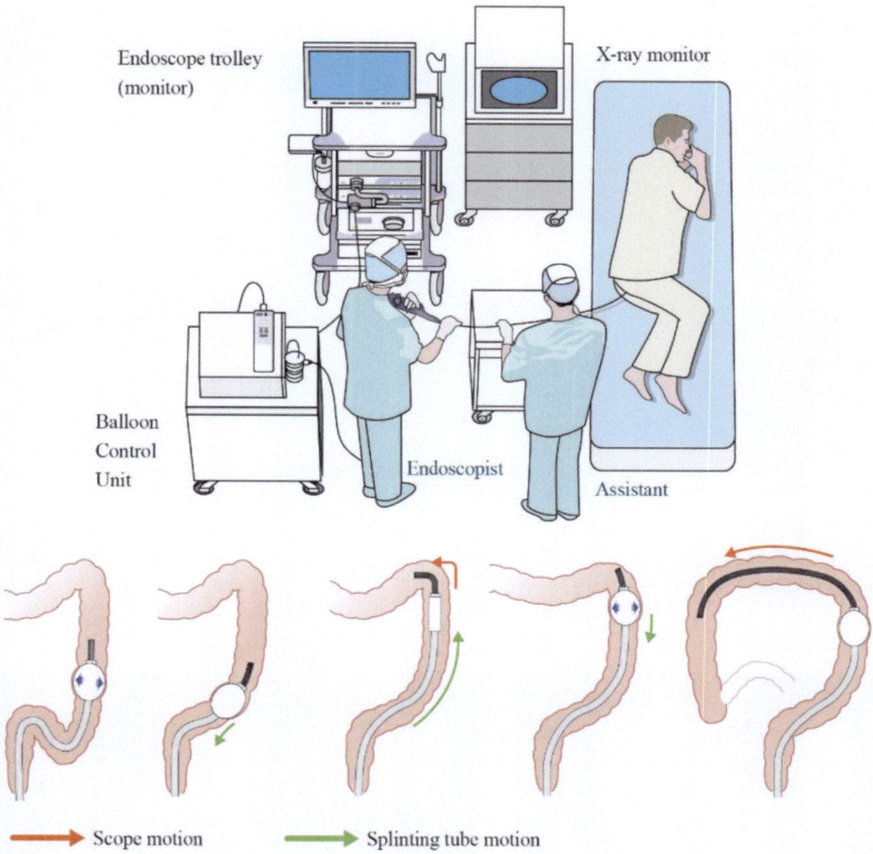

Fig. 3.15 Example of retrograde insertion

the terminal ileum, causing it to slip backward (Fig. 3.16). If looping happens and insertion becomes difficult, changing the patient's position to the left lateral side or applying manual pressure to the right lower abdomen can help reduce the loop and facilitate smoother entry into the terminal ileum.

If insertion remains challenging despite these methods, performing retroflexion in the cecum and pushing the small bowel enteroscope toward the ileocecal valve can help, as the cecum provides support, making entry into the terminal ileum easier (Fig. 3.17).

3.6.4 Deep Insertion Method

For deep insertion, the enteroscope creates a circular loop in the small bowel, which can rotate either clockwise or counterclockwise. During insertion in the proximal small bowel, a combination of both rotations may occur. After the shortening

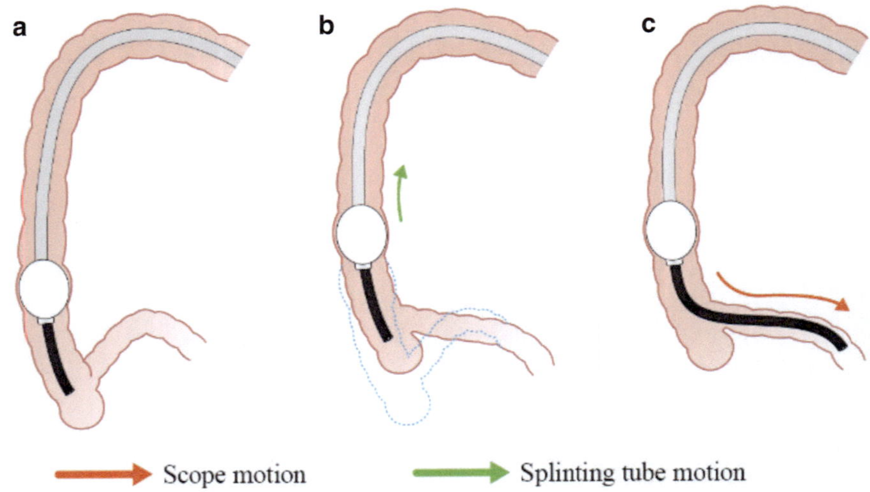

Fig. 3.16 Insertion method into the terminal ileum. ① Inflate the balloon in the ascending colon. ② Withdraw the splinting tube to reduce the insertion angle. ③ Advance the scope past the Bauhin's valve into the ileum

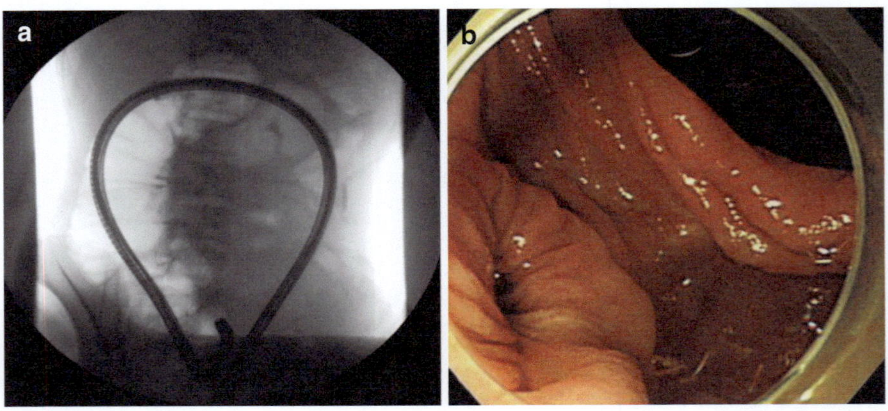

Fig. 3.17 Insertion method into the terminal ileum (retrograde insertion). After retroflexing the endoscope in the cecum, advance it toward the ileocecal valve, as seen in the retroflexed view

procedure, the enteroscope can be rotated either direction. Insertion can be performed regardless of rotation direction; however, clockwise rotation often results in the recurrence of a large intragastric loop when advancing the scope, which can hinder effective deep insertion without unwanted looping (Fig. 3.18a). In contrast, counterclockwise rotation typically does not cause intragastric looping and allows for more effective deep insertion (Fig. 3.18b) [7]. Another potential drawback of

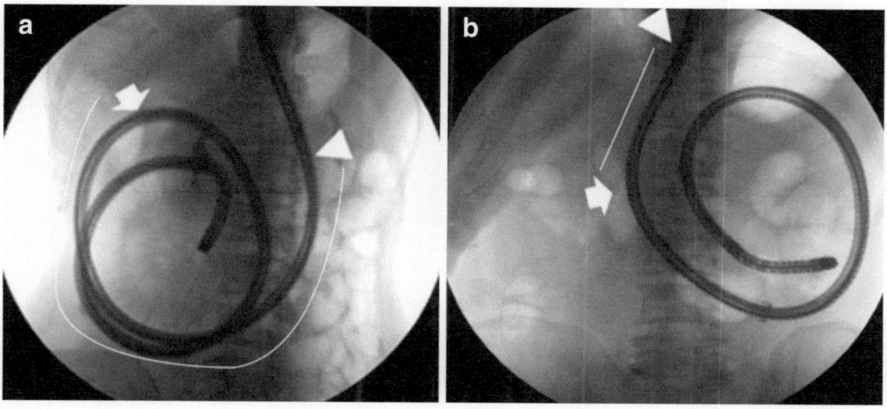

Fig. 3.18 Clockwise or counterclockwise rotation. (**a**) In clockwise rotation, a large intragastric loop recurs when the scope is pushed forward (arrow, pyloric ring; arrowhead, esophagogastric junction). (**b**) In counterclockwise rotation, the intragastric loop is effectively controlled without recurrence during insertion

clockwise rotation is the risk of post-bronchial artery embolization acute pancreatitis, which can result from severe mechanical strain or ischemic injury to the pancreatic body and the tail.

To transmit the pushing force to the distal end of the enteroscope, it is important to avoid sharp angulation during insertion. Sharp angulation often prevents further advancement of the enteroscope, instead stretching the small bowel. Fluoroscopic guidance shows that a more counterclockwise rotation can aid in greater advancement. However, sharp angulation can prevent effective force transfer to the distal end, leading to unnecessary stretching of the bowel. Using contrast dye infusion can help predict the insertion direction. If sharp angulations are encountered, withdrawing the enteroscope and overtube can help straighten the small bowel loop. By visualizing the proximal small bowel with contrast dye, the straightening process can be monitored, allowing the operator to identify the right point to stop shortening and resume advancing the scope (Fig. 3.19).

3.7 Additional Tips for Deep Insertion

3.7.1 Minimizing Backward Slippage of the SBE During Shortening

In SBE, since only one balloon is used, the ability to anchor the bowel is weaker, which increases the likelihood of the distal tip of the enteroscope retracting. As shown in Fig. 3.20, when the enteroscope forms a gentle forward circular loop, attempting to shorten the bowel often results in a backward slippage of the enteroscope.

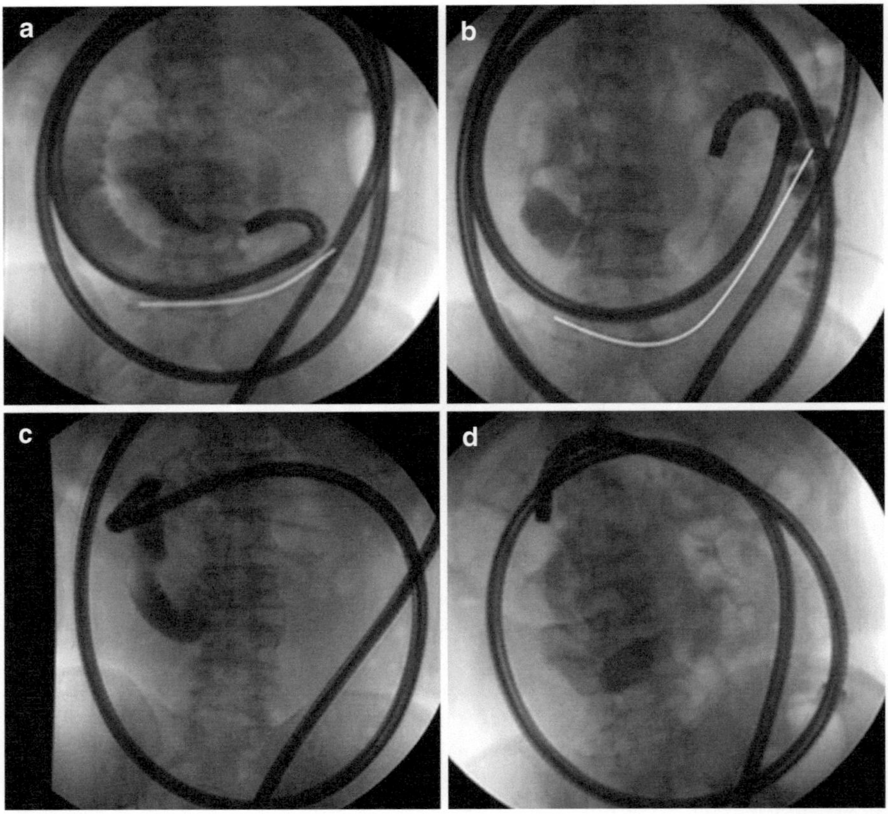

Fig. 3.19 Determining the optimal insertion direction. (**a**) The small bowel loop is angulated in a U-shape around the enteroscope tip, visualized with contrast dye infusion. (**b**) Without straightening the U-shaped loop, pushing the scope results in minimal advancement and insignificant stretching of the small bowel. (**c**) Withdrawing the enteroscope along with the overtube helps straighten the small bowel loop. (**d**) After releasing the angulated enteroscope tip, the enteroscope and the proximal small bowel align in a straight line, effectively transferring the pushing force

To minimize this issue, use the up, down, left, and right knobs or twist the enteroscope shaft to shape the distal tip into a hook (Fig. 3.21). Shortening the bowel while keeping this hooked position helps prevent backward slippage of the tip and ensures effective shortening.

3.7.2 Compression Method

When the proximal small bowel forms an acute angle that cannot be sufficiently straightened through shortening, the compression method, typically used during colonoscopy, can help advance the endoscope. As shown in Fig. 3.22, when the

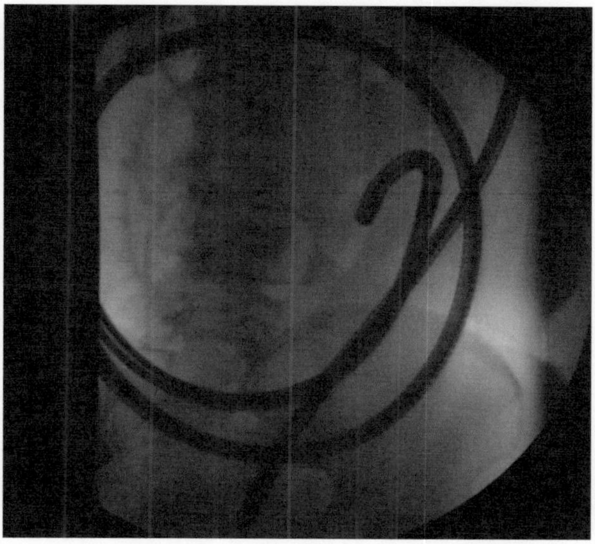

Fig. 3.20 The distal tip of the endoscope frequently slips backward during shortening when a circular loop is formed

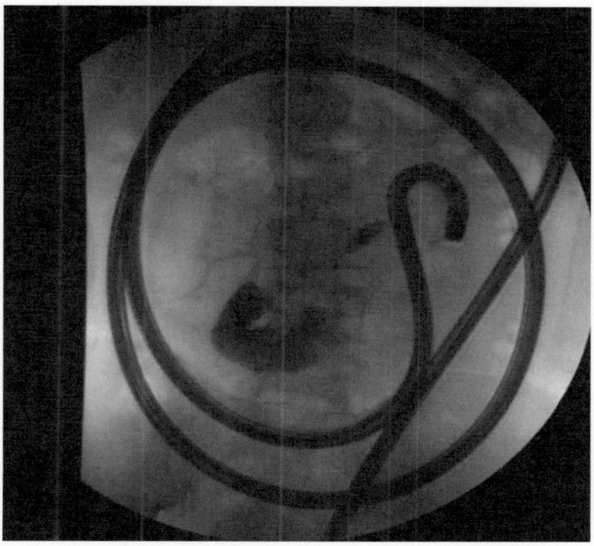

Fig. 3.21 Forming the distal tip into a hook shape to minimize backward slippage of the SBE during shortening

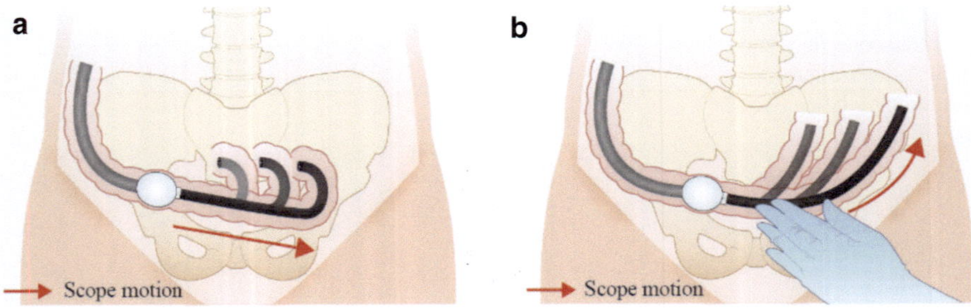

Fig. 3.22 In case (**a**), when the pushing force is not effectively transmitted to the distal tip of the endoscope and only causes unnecessary stretching of the bowel, applying manual pressure as shown in case (**b**) provides support, allowing the pushing force to reach the distal tip of the endoscope effectively

endoscope encounters a sharp angle that hinders progression, applying external compression provides the necessary force to guide the enteroscope into the proximal small bowel.

References

1. Takano N, Yamada A, Watabe H, et al. Single-balloon versus double-balloon endoscopy for achieving total enteroscopy: a randomized, controlled trial. Gastrointest Endosc. 2011;73:734–9.
2. Lenz P, Meister T, Manno M, et al. CO2 insufflation during single-balloon enteroscopy: a multicenter randomized controlled trial. Endoscopy. 2014;46:53–8.
3. Moreels TG, Kouinche Madenko N, et al. Therapeutic enteroscopy using a new single-balloon enteroscope: a case series. Endosc Int Open. 2016;4:E918–21.
4. Li X, Zhao YJ, Dai J, et al. Carbon dioxide insufflation improves the intubation depth and total enteroscopy rate in single-balloon enteroscopy: a randomized, controlled, double-blind trial. Gut. 2014;63:1560–5.
5. Mehdizadeh S, Ross A, Gerson L, et al. What is the learning curve associated with double-balloon enteroscopy? Technical details and early experience in 6 U.S. tertiary care centers. Gastrointest Endosc. 2006;64:740–50.
6. Araki A, Tsuchiya K, Okada E, et al. Single-operator double-balloon endoscopy (DBE) is as effective as dual-operator DBE. J Gastroenterol Hepatol. 2009;24:770–5.
7. Kim J. Training in endoscopy: enteroscopy. Clin Endosc. 2017;50:328–33.

Therapeutic Procedures of Balloon-Assisted Enteroscopy

4

Tomonori Yano, Satoshi Shinozaki, and Hironori Yamamoto

4.1 Therapeutic Endoscopy in the Small Intestine

The small intestine is a long tubular organ located between the stomach and the colon. Unlike the duodenum, the jejunum and the ileum are largely unfixed within the abdominal cavity. Consequently, conventional endoscopy has limited therapeutic utility in the small intestine due to the inability to effectively transmit manipulative force to the scope's distal end. However, the advent of balloon-assisted endoscopy (BAE) has revolutionized small intestinal interventions. The balloon-equipped overtube of the BAE system securely anchors to the intestinal wall, creating fixed points and minimizing intestinal elongation. This enhancement in scope stability enables effective therapeutic endoscopy, even in the deep small intestine, comparable to procedures performed in the stomach or the colon.

4.2 Selection of the Appropriate Scope

Balloon-assisted endoscopy (BAE) comprises two primary types: double-balloon endoscopy (DBE), which features a balloon at the scope tip, and single-balloon endoscopy (SBE), which lacks this feature. Despite these structural differences, the fundamental principles of operation are the same.

Currently available DBE models include:

EN-840 T: Equipped with a water-jet channel, a working channel diameter of 3.2 mm, and a working length of 200 cm.

T. Yano · S. Shinozaki · H. Yamamoto (✉)
Division of Gastroenterology, Department of Medicine, Jichi Medical University, Tochigi, Japan
e-mail: ireef@jichi.ac.jp

J.-J. Park et al. (eds.), *Balloon-Assisted Enteroscopy*,
https://doi.org/10.1007/978-981-95-2445-7_4

EN-580XP: Features a 2.2-mm working channel diameter and a working length of 200 cm.

EI-580BT: Provides a 3.2-mm working channel diameter and a working length of 155 cm.

Currently available SBE models include:

SIF-H190: Offers a 3.2-mm working channel diameter and a working length of 200 cm.

SIF-H290S: Has a 3.2-mm working channel diameter and a working length of 152 cm.

The differences in working length influence the accessible range within the small intestine, the types of therapeutic devices that can be used, and the time required for device insertion and withdrawal. The working channel diameter also dictates the choice of devices. For example, while a 2.2-mm channel accommodates injection needles and small-diameter snares, it cannot support the use of clips or dilation balloons. Therefore, selecting the appropriate scope requires consideration of the target lesion and the devices needed for the procedure. Additionally, many BAE scopes other than the DBE scope of EN-840 T do not have a dedicated water-jet channel. To perform injection or contrast studies while a therapeutic device is inserted through the working channel, alternative techniques are necessary. For instance, replacing the standard forceps valve with the BioShield® Irrigator (US Endoscopy; Fig. 4.1) enables the injection of liquids through the remaining space in the working channel while maintaining the device in position.

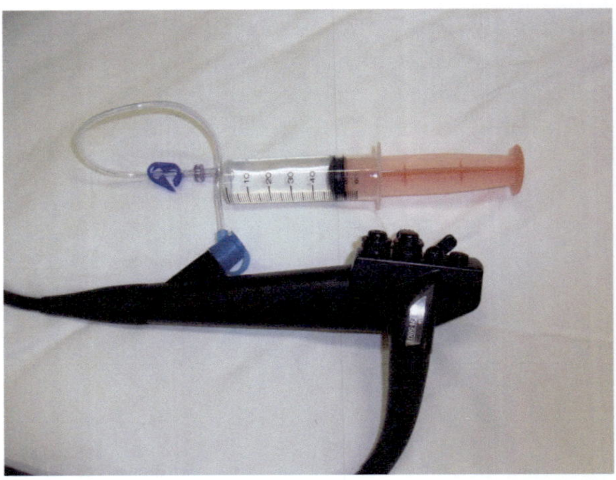

Fig. 4.1 BioShield irrigator

4.3 Selection of the Appropriate Hood

Compared to other parts of the gastrointestinal tract, the small intestine has a narrower lumen and more frequent angulations, which can hinder adequate visualization during endoscopy. This challenge can be mitigated by attaching an appropriate hood to the tip of the BAE scope.

For hemostatic procedures and polypectomy, a cylindrical hood with a length of 4 mm is recommended. Suitable options include the Disposable Distal Attachment D-201-10704 (Olympus, Tokyo, Japan; Fig. 4.2a) or the Space Adjuster (TOP Co.、 Tokyo, Japan; Fig. 4.2b). These hoods not only facilitate visualization but also maintain an optimal working distance from the lesion. This allows effective compression hemostasis using the hood's lateral surface and improves visualization of the stalk in pedunculated polyps. Additionally, a clip can be safely deployed and held in the internal space of the hood, preventing injury to the intestinal wall during the scope manipulation. A cylindrical hood is also beneficial in techniques such as the Crossed-clip Strangulation Method, which is discussed later.

For stricture dilation, the CAST hood (TOP Co.), a thin, tapered hood with measurement markings, is preferred. The specific advantages of this hood will be described in subsequent sections.

4.4 Hemostatic Procedures

4.4.1 Selection of Insertion Route

For cases of overt ongoing bleeding, characterized by continuous macroscopic hematochezia or melena, the oral route is preferred without prior bowel preparation. In the small intestine, retrograde flow of intestinal fluid is minimal due to peristalsis. Thus, encountering bloody intestinal fluid during oral insertion suggests proximity to the bleeding source. In contrast, insertion via the anal route even with adequate

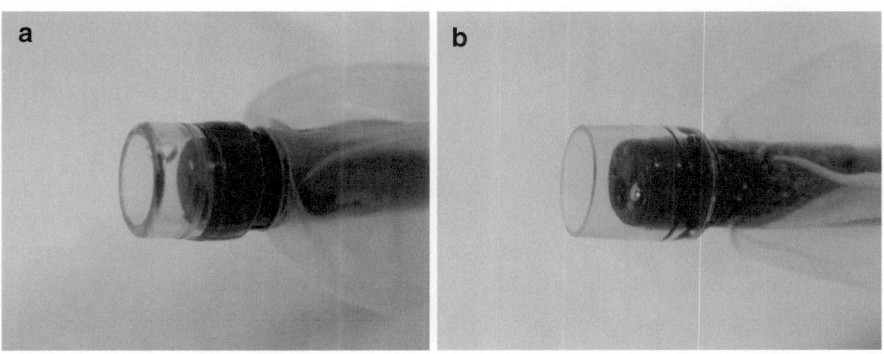

Fig. 4.2 (**a**) Cylindrical hood (D-201-10704, OLYMPUS). (**b**) Cylindrical hood (Space Adjuster, TOP)

bowel preparation, scope insertion is challenging in a visual field obstructed by bloody fluid and clots. Moreover, the retrograde flow of bloody fluid caused by insufflation can hinder the identification of the bleeding site. However, if pre-procedural imaging indicates that the bleeding source is located in the distal ileum, the anal route should be considered, as reaching this area may be challenging via the oral route.

In cases of occult bleeding, characterized by persistent positive fecal occult blood tests and iron-deficiency anemia, or in previous overt bleeding where macroscopic bleeding is no longer present at the time of endoscopy, the route closest to the suspected lesion should be selected based on pre-procedural findings.

When no clues regarding the lesion location are available and a complete small bowel evaluation is desired, the anal route is typically prioritized due to its lower patient burden and reduced risk of complications such as acute pancreatitis. During this anal approach, the endoscopist inserts the scope as deeply as possible, marking the deepest reached point with dye or clips. Subsequently, the oral route is used to advance the scope to the marked point, achieving total enteroscopy.

4.4.2 Considerations for the Oral Route

When performing BAE via the oral route, the procedure is conducted with the patient in the left lateral decubitus position, as in upper gastrointestinal endoscopy. The BAE technique achieves deep small bowel access by shortening the bowel during the procedure, folding the proximal intestine onto the overtube with a balloon. This shortening maneuver increases intraluminal pressure in the proximal intestine, potentially inducing vomiting and increasing the risk of aspiration pneumonia.

To minimize this risk, gastric contents should be thoroughly suctioned as soon as the scope enters the stomach to ensure that there is minimal material available for regurgitation. Additionally, insufflation should be minimized, even when using carbon dioxide, to prevent excessive increase in intraluminal pressure.

During oral insertion, the detection of bloody intestinal fluid suggests proximity to the bleeding source. Unlike other parts of the gastrointestinal tract, the small intestine lacks clear anatomical landmarks. If excessive washing is performed, the area of interest may be lost, complicating the search for the bleeding source. To avoid this, place a clip at the site of bloody intestinal fluid before initiating washing, establishing a landmark for further investigation.

Progressing further, the endoscopist should monitor the characteristics of the bloody fluid. If the fluid becomes dark red, it is likely that the bleeding source has been passed. In this case, place two clips to mark this point. The bleeding source is then assumed to be located between the single-clip site and the double-clip site. Focused investigation within this marked range can efficiently identify the bleeding source.

4.4.3 Considerations for the Anal Route

When performing BAE via the anal route, the procedure begins with the patient in the left lateral decubitus position, similar to lower gastrointestinal endoscopy. Positional adjustments are made as needed during insertion. In patients with active small bowel bleeding, the presence of bloody intestinal fluid or blood clots can obstruct the visual field and necessitate increased insufflation during insertion. Excessive insufflation not only reduces insertion efficiency but also pushes bloody intestinal fluid proximally, making it harder to localize the bleeding source based on its distribution. To address these challenges, visualization can be maintained using the gel immersion technique, which is described later. This method minimizes increase in intraluminal pressure and prevents the proximal displacement of bloody intestinal fluid, aiding in the identification of the bleeding source.

In cases where extravasation is identified in the ileum on contrast-enhanced computed tomography (CT), the estimated distance from the ileocecal valve to the bleeding site should be calculated preoperatively. During BAE, once the scope reaches the estimated location, it is advisable to place a clip as a marker for further guidance in identifying and treating the bleeding source.

4.4.4 Visualization with Gel Immersion Endoscopy

For effective endoscopic hemostasis, precise localization of the bleeding site is essential. However, the narrow lumen of the small intestine, compared to other segments of the gastrointestinal tract, is prone to rapid occlusion by bloody intestinal fluid. In cases of ongoing bleeding, suctioning the bloody fluid often results in its rapid reaccumulation. While submersion in water can sometimes aid in locating the bleeding site, high-volume bleeding quickly mixes with water, reducing visualization quality. To address this limitation, the gel immersion endoscopy technique has been developed, using transparent gel instead of water [1].

Viscoclear® (Otsuka Pharmaceutical Factory, Tokushima, Japan) is a transparent gel with appropriate viscosity for maintaining visualization in gastrointestinal endoscopy. It can be easily introduced through the working channel of the scope. Unlike water, the gel does not immediately mix with bloody fluid, creating a transparent field around the scope's tip. The additional gel can be injected through the working channel as needed to maintain this transparent space while searching for the bleeding site. Once identified, hemostasis can be achieved using hemostatic clips.

Key considerations for effective use:

1. Scope and accessories:
   Use a scope with a working channel diameter of at least 2.8 mm (preferably 3.2 mm) to facilitate gel injection while a hemostatic clip is inserted. Employ the BioShield® Irrigator (US Endoscopy, OH, USA) as the forceps valve and attach a cylindrical hood to the scope tip.

2. Preparation:
   Before injecting the gel, aspirate excess gas to collapse the lumen. Inject 100–150 mL of gel into the space between the intestinal wall and blood clots, rather than the center of the lumen. For DBE, inflating the balloon at the scope tip prevents backflow of the gel and allows for gel retention. To avoid fixing the scope to the intestinal wall, partially deflate the balloon and hold it in a semi-inflated state using the "PAUSE" button.
3. Precautions during use:
   (i) Avoid insufflation entirely, as bubbles hinder visualization and are difficult to eliminate.
   (ii) Refrain from suctioning until hemostasis is achieved, as this can reintroduce bloody fluid into the field.
   (iii) When removing instruments, do so slowly while simultaneously injecting additional gel through the BioShield® Irrigator to maintain the clear field.

Gel immersion endoscopy is particularly useful during the anal route insertion in cases with poor bowel preparation or active bleeding. After aspirating excess gas, press the cylindrical hood against the intestinal wall and inject gel, filling the space within the hood with transparent gel. Gradually inject small amounts of gel between the hood and the intestinal wall, using the folds as visual landmarks for scope insertion. This method allows for insertion with low intraluminal pressure, minimizing proximal displacement of bloody fluid and facilitating identification of the bleeding source [2].

Gel immersion endoscopy is not limited to small bowel bleeding but is also effective in managing other gastrointestinal hemorrhages. It is particularly useful when bloody fluid or residual material obscures the bleeding site.

4.4.5 Hemostatic Methods Based on Lesion Type

4.4.5.1 Vascular Lesions

Gastrointestinal vascular lesions, excluding distinct pathologies such as varices and hemangiomas, can be histologically classified into three types:

1. Lesions with characteristics of veins and capillaries (angioectasia).
2. Lesions with characteristics of arteries (Dieulafoy's lesion).
3. Lesions with characteristics of both arteries and veins (arteriovenous malformation, (AVM)).

To select appropriate therapeutic strategies, the presence or absence of arterial components (e.g., pulsatility) is evaluated using the Yano-Yamamoto classification of small intestinal vascular lesions (Fig. 4.3) [3], which categorizes lesions into six types:

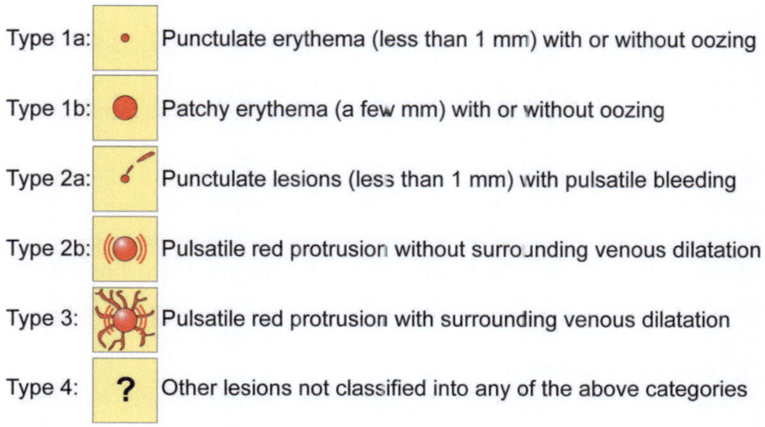

Fig. 4.3 Endoscopic classification of vascular lesions of the small intestine (Yano-Yamamoto classification)

Type 1a: Punctate (<1 mm) erythema with or without oozing.
Type 1b: Patchy (a few mm) erythema with or without oozing.
Type 2a: Punctate lesion (<1 mm) with pulsatile bleeding.
Type 2b: Pulsatile red protrusion without surrounding venous dilatation.
Type 3: Pulsatile red protrusion with surrounding venous dilatation.
Type 4: Other lesions not classified into any of the above categories.

Type 1 Lesions
These correspond to angioectasia (1) and can vary in size and distribution, often appearing as multiple lesions within the same patient. They may present with overt bleeding or anemia, but many cases are asymptomatic. Treatment typically involves argon plasma coagulation (APC) or, in cases with few lesions, cold snaring followed by clipping without electrocautery [4].

Type 2 Lesions
These correspond to Dieulafoy's lesions (2) and are characterized by arterial features, including an internal elastic lamina. The arterial nature makes the blood vessels less visible when not actively bleeding, rendering non-bleeding type 2a lesions difficult to detect. Type 2b lesions appear as small, slightly reddened, pulsatile protrusions and require careful observation. Both subtypes are treated by ligation of the causative vessel with hemostatic clips.

Type 3 Lesions
These correspond to AVM (3) and feature pulsatile red protrusion with surrounding venous dilatation, suggesting arteriovenous shunting. Small lesions may be treated with clip application to feeding vessels. However, larger lesions often require transcatheter arterial embolization or surgical intervention.

Type 4 Lesions

Atypical lesions with unique morphology that cannot be classified are designated as type 4. These cases require further evaluation, including endoscopic ultrasound (EUS) or other diagnostic modalities, to determine an appropriate treatment plan.

4.4.5.2 Inflammatory Lesions

Inflammatory lesions, such as ulcers or erosions, may require tissue biopsy or culture tests to identify the underlying disease and guide medical therapy. When exposed vessels are identified at the ulcer base, hemostatic clips should be used for treatment.

4.4.5.3 Tumorous Lesions

Tumorous lesions may be amenable to endoscopic treatments such as polypectomy or ligation using detachable snares. However, cases often require surgical resection or chemotherapy, depending on the lesion's malignancy and progression.

4.4.6 In Case the Bleeding Source Cannot Be Identified

Emergency BAE for active small intestinal bleeding has a higher likelihood of identifying the bleeding source compared to procedures performed after spontaneous hemostasis. However, even during emergency BAE, it is possible to encounter fresh blood clots without successfully identifying the bleeding source.

In such cases, the bleeding may have originated from a type 2a lesion in the Yano-Yamamoto classification of small intestinal vascular lesions [3], corresponding to a Dieulafoy's lesion. These lesions are notoriously difficult to detect once spontaneous hemostasis occurs, as their arterial characteristics and punctate nature make them inconspicuous when not actively bleeding.

To address this, patients and their families should be thoroughly informed of the possibility of rebleeding and instructed to seek emergency care immediately if rebleeding occurs. Close and careful follow-up is essential to ensure timely intervention in case of recurrence.

4.5 Polyp Treatment

4.5.1 Thin Wall of the Small Intestine

The small intestine has a thinner wall than the colon, making it essential to avoid perforation while treating small intestinal polyps. For small, flat polyps, cold snare polypectomy (CSP), which involves resection without electrocautery, is safer. For lesions too large for CSP, submucosal injection can be performed to avoid involving the muscular layer, followed by snare resection (endoscopic mucosal resection (EMR)). Alternatively, the snare can be tightened under water immersion before a brief application of electrocautery for resection (underwater EMR), with closure using clips to prevent complications.

For lesions larger than 2 cm, endoscopic submucosal dissection (ESD) may be necessary. However, ESD in the small intestine, particularly in the duodenum, carries a high risk of perforation and bleeding. To mitigate this risk, the Pocket Creation Method (PCM) is recommended, as it allows precise dissection, leaving a thin layer of the submucosa intact [5].

4.5.2 Mild Intussusception Mimicking Pedunculated Polyps

The small intestine is highly mobile within the abdominal cavity, with a narrow lumen and a thin wall, making it prone to intussusception. Polyps larger than 15 mm may cause intussusception, and even smaller polyps can collectively form the leading edge. In mild intussusception, the muscularis propria may be pulled inward, appearing as a pedunculated polyp with a thick stalk on endoscopy. If a snare is placed on what appears to be the stalk and resection is performed, the muscularis propria may be inadvertently cut, leading to perforation (Fig. 4.4). When encountering a pedunculated polyp with a thick stalk, the possibility of intussusception should be considered. It is safer to retract the polyp proximally before snaring closer to the polyp rather than at the stalk's base to avoid cutting the muscularis propria.

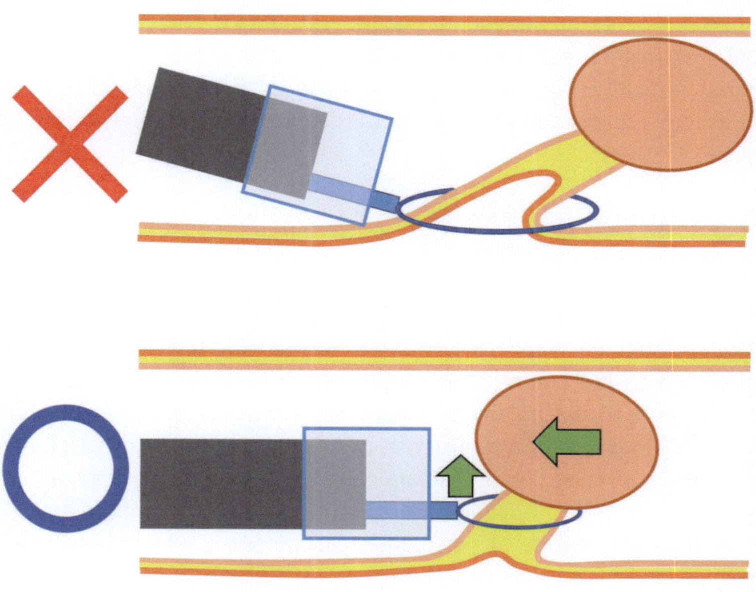

Fig. 4.4 Pseudo-pedunculated polyp

4.5.3 Techniques for Reducing Intussusception

1. For short-segment intussusception:
   In antegrade BAE, suction can be used to pull the polyp into the hood and move it proximally, reducing the intussusception.
   In retrograde BAE, the polyp can be pushed proximally using the hood to reduce the intussusception.
2. For long-segment intussusception:

   In oral DBE, the intussuscepted segment can be carefully traversed, followed by inflation of the scope-tip balloon. Retracting the scope while the balloon is semi-inflated can reduce the intussusception.
   In anal DBE, the scope-tip balloon can be inflated near the intussuscepted segment, and contrast medium can be gradually injected through the working channel to push the intussusception proximally, achieving reduction [6].

4.6 Small Intestinal Polyps in Familial Adenomatous Polyposis

4.6.1 Characteristics of Familial Adenomatous Polyposis

Familial adenomatous polyposis (FAP) is characterized by the presence of innumerable adenomas in the colon, which necessitates total colectomy to prevent malignancy. However, 50–70% of patients also develop adenomas in the small intestine, with a high prevalence in the duodenum. Patients with extensive duodenal involvement often exhibit lesions extending into the jejunum [7]. In addition to the duodenum and proximal jejunum, polyps frequently develop in the ileal pouch after total colectomy. Typically, flat lesions are numerous in the duodenum, decreasing in number as they progress into the jejunum. Adenomas are also common in the duodenal papilla.

4.6.2 Treatment of Polyps

Because small polyps have a lower malignant potential, some argue that treatment should be deferred until they exceed 10 mm in size [8]. However, leaving multiple small polyps untreated can result in coalescence into larger lesions, increasing the difficulty of endoscopic treatment, sometimes requiring endoscopic submucosal dissection (ESD) [9], with a higher risk of adverse events. Post-colectomy adhesions can also complicate surgical treatment. For polyps smaller than 10 mm, cold snare polypectomy (CSP) is recommended. This method, widely used for colorectal polyps, minimizes the risk of perforation and bleeding while allowing efficient treatment of multiple lesions in a short time [10, 11]. When performing CSP on multiple polyps consecutively, using a scope with a large working channel diameter combined with a thin snare allows for suction-based retrieval of resected specimens without removing the snare. Incorporating the BioShield® irrigator enables washing without removing the snare, further enhancing procedural efficiency.

For polyps measuring 10–20 mm, underwater EMR is the preferred approach. For polyps larger than 20 mm, ESD is the ideal approach [12]. Considering the balance of risks and benefits, when it is challenging to perform ESD, treatment with planned piecemeal underwater EMR is an alternative option for large lesions with no malignant findings.

4.6.3 Post-Treatment Follow-Up

The development and growth rate of small intestinal polyps in FAP vary among individuals, necessitating treatment intervals tailored to each patient, ranging from every 6 months to 2 years. While most lesions occur in the duodenum, focusing solely on the proximal duodenum with standard esophagogastroduodenoscopy can lead to undetected and untreated larger lesions in the distal duodenum or the jejunum [9]. Therefore, comprehensive evaluation and treatment of the entire duodenum and proximal jejunum are crucial during follow-up.

4.7 Small Intestinal Polyps in Peutz-Jeghers Syndrome

4.7.1 Characteristics of Peutz-Jeghers Syndrome

Peutz-Jeghers syndrome (PJS) is characterized by mucocutaneous pigmentation on the lips, oral cavity, and fingertips, as well as the presence of multiple polyps throughout the gastrointestinal tract, excluding the esophagus. While these polyps are predominantly hamartomatous, larger lesions carry a potential risk of malignancy. In addition, PJS is associated with an increased risk of extra-gastrointestinal malignancies, including lung, breast, pancreatic, and cervical malignancies, requiring regular surveillance in adulthood.

Clinically, the most concerning complication is intestinal intussusception, often requiring emergency surgery. Many patients experience intussusception in their teenage years, resulting in open abdominal surgery. However, once abdominal surgery is performed, intra-abdominal adhesions often develop, which can limit the reach of balloon-assisted endoscopy (BAE). If polyps develop in segments of the small intestine that are inaccessible via BAE, repeat surgery may be required, perpetuating a vicious cycle. Multiple partial small bowel resections over a lifetime may result in short bowel syndrome. To prevent such complications, surveillance of the small intestine should be started before the age of 8, even if the patient is asymptomatic, and polyps that could cause intussusception should be treated with BAE. In cases where patients experience symptoms such as abdominal pain or anemia before the age of 8, total enteroscopy and BAE-based treatment should be conducted regardless of age [13].

Adverse events associated with treating PJS-related small intestinal polyps using BAE include intussusception, acute pancreatitis, perforation, and bleeding. Among these, perforation necessitating surgical intervention is of particular concern, as it exacerbates intra-abdominal adhesions and compromises the feasibility of future BAE procedures. Every effort should be made to avoid perforation during treatment.

4.7.2 Perform Retrograde BAE First

In PJS, small intestinal polyps are more commonly distributed in the duodenum and the jejunum than in the ileum. However, retrograde BAE is recommended first.

If anterograde BAE is performed first, resected polyps may become lodged against distal polyps during peristalsis, potentially causing intussusception. To mitigate this risk, retrograde BAE should be performed first to treat ileal polyps, followed by antegrade BAE to address duodenal and jejunal polyps.

As part of the bowel preparation for retrograde BAE, CT enterography can be performed by administering a bowel-cleansing agent prior to abdominal dynamic contrast-enhanced CT. This enables visualization of the distribution of large polyps before initiating BAE.

The risk of acute pancreatitis increases when the duration of antegrade BAE exceeds 2 hours. To minimize procedure time for antegrade BAE, retrograde BAE should aim for the deepest possible insertion without time constraints. Mark the deepest reached point with clips or other markers, which can serve as the target endpoint for antegrade BAE, thereby reducing the overall procedure time and associated complications.

4.7.3 Ischemic Treatment as a Safe Option

Polyps in Peutz-Jeghers syndrome (PJS) are often pedunculated or semi-pedunculated and can grow to several centimeters in size. In the narrow lumen of the small intestine, such large polyps can occupy significant space, making it difficult to visualize the entire lesion or capture it entirely with a snare. Even with a cylindrical hood, large blind spots can occur behind the polyp, increasing the risk of unintentionally snaring the intestinal wall and causing perforation. Additionally, pedunculated polyps often have relatively large blood vessels within the stalk, posing a risk of intraoperative and postoperative bleeding if resected. Although pathological evaluation of lesions requires their resection and retrieval, this necessity is relatively low for PJS polyps, which are predominantly hamartomas. Therefore, ischemic treatment using detachable snares or clips to occlude blood flow of the stalk, causing necrosis and natural detachment of the polyp, is a viable alternative [14].

Ischemic treatment theoretically minimizes the risks of bleeding and perforation. Additionally, clipping the stalk does not require full visualization of the lesion, making it a practical and time-efficient option, even in challenging conditions such as adhesions or angulated sections of the intestine. After blood flow to the polyp is occluded, it typically turns purple within seconds and undergoes necrosis, detaching naturally within hours to a few days. During this period, dark red stools may be observed, indicating necrotic polyps and that ischemic treatment is effective. As long as the anemia does not worsen, observation is sufficient, and no further intervention is necessary.

4.7.4 Ischemic Treatment with Clips Underwater

The ischemic treatment described earlier can be performed using clips for pedunculated or semi-pedunculated polyps with stalk diameters approximately equal to the length of the clip. At our institution, EZ Clip Long (HX-610-090 L, Olympus) is used for this purpose. Applying a clip to the stalk of a pedunculated polyp is relatively straightforward if the polyp naturally hangs down due to gravity. However, when the polyp lies flat, securing the clip becomes challenging. This issue can be addressed by performing the procedure underwater, as the polyp floats in water, improving visualization of the stalk and facilitating clip placement. Therefore, it is recommended to perform the entire procedure, from endoscopic insertion into the small intestine to the completion of the examination, under water immersion using the water exchange method (described in Sect. 4.8.8). Most polyps require only a single clip for effective ischemia, turning purple within seconds. However, in some cases, a single clip may not fully occlude blood flow, and the polyp does not change color. In such instances, the Crossed-clip Strangulation Method [15] can be employed to add a second clip (Fig. 4.5). In this method, the first clip is displaced laterally using the tip of the cylindrical hood, altering the orientation of the stalk. The second clip is then applied in a direction approximately 90 degrees different from the first. This crosswise application of two clips ensures stronger occlusion of blood flow, enhancing the effectiveness of the ischemic treatment.

4.7.5 Ischemic Treatment with Detachable Snares

For semi-pedunculated polyps without a distinct stalk, or pedunculated polyps with stalks too thick for clips, ischemic treatment using a detachable snare [16] is recommended. Detachable snares are made of polyamide, which is less rigid than conventional metal snares, making it challenging to encircle large lesions in the narrow lumen of the small intestine. Underwater procedures can further narrow the intestinal lumen, so insufflation may be necessary to expand the lumen and facilitate snare placement. Most polyps treated with a detachable snare undergo necrosis and detach naturally. However, in large polyps with thick stalks, ischemic treatment may result in partial shrinkage, causing the ligation to loosen and the polyp to persist.

In such cases, the excess loop of the detachable snare should be preserved rather than cut. For additional treatment, a clip can be applied near the stopper on the excess loop, which can then be grasped with forceps and pulled into the working

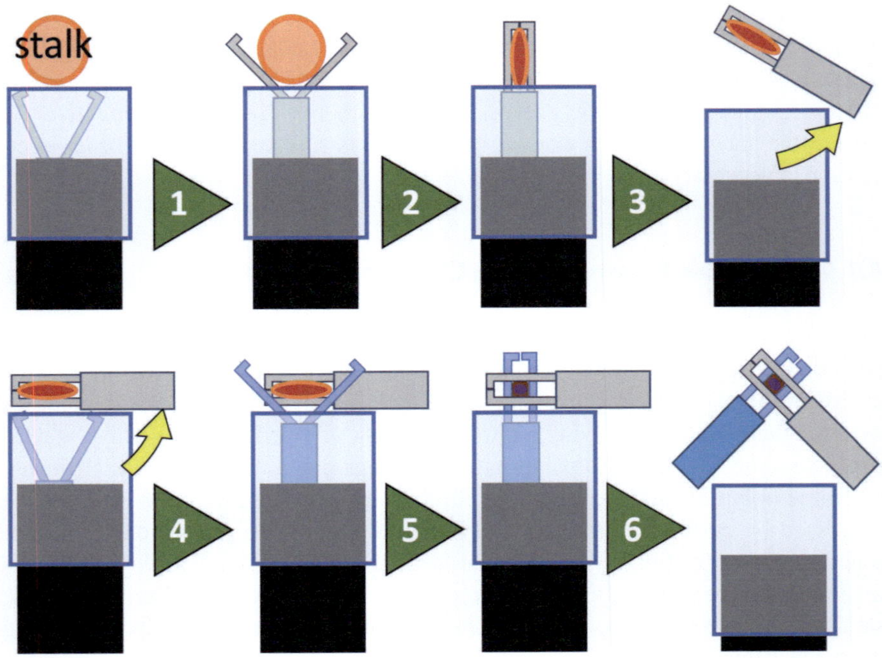

Fig. 4.5 Crossed-clip strangulation

channel. The clip remains outside the working channel, pressing against the stopper to tighten the loop further, achieving effective ligation [17]. This approach provides a reliable method to manage large, challenging polyps that are resistant to initial ischemic treatment, ensuring effective and safe outcomes.

4.7.6 Giant Polyps Unsuitable for Detachable Snares

In some cases, polyps in Peutz-Jeghers syndrome (PJS) grow so large that even the largest detachable snares (maximum diameter 30 mm) cannot encircle them. These giant polyps often have thick stalks, making it difficult to achieve sufficient blood flow occlusion with even two clips. For such polyps, multiple clips can be applied to the stalk from various angles to reduce blood flow. Following this, piecemeal resection with a snare can be attempted. It is not necessary to remove the entire polyp in a single session. Once the lesion is reduced in size through piecemeal resection, a detachable snare can be applied to the base of the stalk to occlude blood flow. Giant polyps also carry a higher risk of malignancy. Therefore, whenever feasible, resected specimens should be retrieved for pathological evaluation.

PJS polyps often exhibit branched structures, which can interfere with the placement of a detachable snare. In such cases, clips can be applied to the base of the branches to induce necrosis and detachment. Once the branches are eliminated, a detachable snare can be safely applied to the main lesion for definitive treatment. This staged approach minimizes risks and ensures effective management of complex giant polyps.

4.7.7 Treatment During Insertion and Additional Treatment During Withdrawal

Using the water exchange method (described in Sect. 4.8.8), ischemic treatment can be performed during insertion without significantly worsening insertion conditions. Treating large polyps with ischemic methods during insertion allows for monitoring color changes in the polyps during withdrawal. If necessary, additional treatment can be applied during the withdrawal phase, ensuring comprehensive and effective management of the lesions.

4.7.8 In Case That Complete Small Bowel Observation Is Not Possible

In Peutz-Jeghers syndrome (PJS), many patients have a history of open abdominal surgery, leading to intra-abdominal adhesions. As a result, even with bidirectional BAE, complete observation of the small intestine may not be feasible. Fortunately, PJS polyps are typically concentrated in the proximal and distal segments of the small intestine, with relatively few polyps occurring in the middle portion. However, over time, polyps can develop in the midsection as well.

To address this limitation:

1. Place clips as markers at the deepest point reached during retrograde BAE. During antegrade BAE, inject contrast medium at the deepest point reached to check for gross lesions. The use of water immersion during insertion ensures optimal contrast imaging.
2. Alternatively, mark the deepest points reached during both antegrade and retrograde BAE with dye, and use capsule endoscopy to examine the segment between the two marked points.

If polyps are identified in areas inaccessible to BAE, immediate surgical intervention or intraoperative endoscopy is usually unnecessary. Intussusception is less likely to occur in fixed intestinal segments affected by adhesions. In such cases, consider the following strategies:

1. Postpone treatment for approximately 1 year [18], allowing an experienced endoscopist to attempt treatment or use a small-caliber diagnostic scope for therapeutic intervention [19].
2. Address inaccessible polyps during surgical treatment for other malignancies, as PJS patients are at increased risk for cancers in various organs.

This approach prioritizes patient safety and ensures effective management of PJS-related polyps while minimizing unnecessary surgical risks.

4.7.9 Post-treatment Follow-Up

During initial treatment, prioritize larger polyps that are more likely to cause intussusception. The primary objective is to treat all polyps larger than 10 mm. Once this goal is achieved, focus on polyps measuring 5 mm or larger. While PJS-related polyps continue to develop throughout a patient's lifetime, the rate of polyp formation and growth varies significantly among individuals. Some patients may require annual BAE, while other patients may only need it every 5 years. The interval between procedures should be adjusted based on the findings of each BAE session to ensure effective and tailored follow-up care.

4.8 Stricture Dilation

4.8.1 Indications for Stricture Dilation

Endoscopic balloon dilation (EBD) is indicated for a variety of gastrointestinal strictures, including those caused by Crohn's disease, Behçet's disease, Non-steroidal anti-inflammatory drug (NSAID)-associated enteropathy, chronic enteropathy associated with *SLCO2A1* gene (CEAS), ischemic enteritis, and scar strictures following lymphoma chemotherapy. Among these, Crohn's disease-related strictures are the most common in clinical practice; hence, this section focuses on gastrointestinal strictures in Crohn's disease.

Strictures in Crohn's disease are classified as inflammatory or fibrotic. Inflammatory strictures are caused by swelling of the intestinal wall due to active inflammation and can often be improved with medical therapy. In contrast, fibrotic strictures, which develop after inflammation subsides, are the primary indication for EBD. The specific indications for EBD are as follows:

1. Strictures causing symptomatic obstruction.
2. Strictures associated with proximal intestinal dilation.
3. Strictures obstructing endoscopic evaluation or treatment.

EBD is contraindicated in the following situations:

1. Strictures longer than 5 cm.
2. Strictures with severe angulation, deep ulcers, fistulas, fissures, abscesses, or associated malignancy.

4.8.2 Significance of Stricture Dilation in Crohn's Disease

The presence of small intestinal strictures significantly impacts the quality of life by causing symptoms of bowel obstruction. Traditionally, surgical treatment was the only option due to the difficulty of performing endoscopic interventions in the deep small intestine. However, in cases of small intestinal strictures caused by chronic inflammatory bowel diseases such as Crohn's disease, surgical intervention does not cure the underlying disease.

Repeated cycles of disease recurrence, stricture formation, and small bowel resection can ultimately lead to short bowel syndrome, severely affecting patient outcomes. Endoscopic balloon dilation (EBD) offers a minimally invasive alternative, enabling the avoidance or delay of surgical treatment. As a result, EBD is becoming increasingly standardized as a low-risk therapeutic option for small intestinal strictures in Crohn's disease.

4.8.3 Timing of EBD

EBD should be performed during the remission phase of Crohn's disease. However, even when clinical remission is achieved and inflammatory markers are negative, residual ulcers are frequently observed during small bowel endoscopy. Ideally, EBD should be performed during endoscopic remission, characterized by mucosal healing. To achieve this state, remission induction therapy should be intensified with treatments such as corticosteroids, immunomodulators, biologics, or nutritional therapy using elemental diets.

It is important to note that remission induction therapy can lead to the healing of longitudinal ulcers, which may result in the development of strictures. Therefore, dietary adjustments should be implemented to prevent obstruction until the absence of strictures is confirmed with BAE or all identified strictures are managed with EBD.

Approximately 4–6 months after initiation of remission induction therapy, BAE should be performed to assess disease status. If strictures meeting the criteria for EBD are identified, the procedure should be performed at this time.

4.8.4 Insertion Routes for BAE

BAE can be performed via either the oral or the anal route. In Crohn's disease, small intestinal strictures are predominantly located in the ileum, making the anal route more commonly used. However, severe ileal deformation caused by the disease can sometimes make it difficult to reach the stricture site via the anal route. In such cases, the oral route may be attempted. Although the distance to the stricture site is greater with oral insertion, the lesser impact of intestinal deformation may allow easier access to the target. When multiple strictures are distributed throughout a large portion of the small intestine, treating all strictures with EBD via a single route may not be feasible. In such situations, the deepest point reached during the first route can be marked with a clip, and the second route can then be used to access and treat the remaining strictures.

4.8.5 Preparation

Food residues frequently accumulate proximal to the site of a stricture. To address this, dietary intake should be limited to liquid diets or elemental diets starting 1 or 2 days before the procedure. Additionally, sustained-release 5-ASA medications should be temporarily discontinued during this period. For anal-route insertion, bowel preparation requires careful planning to avoid exacerbating symptoms of the stricture. Administering two liters of bowel cleansing agent on the morning of the procedure is not advisable, as it may aggravate stricture-related symptoms. Instead, one liter of bowel preparation agent can be taken in the afternoon of the day before the procedure, followed by another liter on the morning of the procedure. Additional doses may be used as needed. However, in the presence of strictures, achieving perfect bowel preparation is unlikely regardless of the amount administered. It is important to accept some compromise in bowel preparation quality while ensuring patient safety and procedural feasibility.

4.8.6 Use of the CAST Hood

Small intestinal strictures in Crohn's disease are often eccentric and accompanied by intestinal deformation, making it difficult to obtain a direct frontal view of the stricture. Additionally, due to the design of the endoscope, the objective lens and the working channel are positioned separately. As a result, even if the stricture is visualized on the screen, passing a guidewire through it can be challenging. When attempting to insert the guidewire from a close distance, alignment issues occur, while at a greater distance, visualizing or accurately targeting the stricture becomes difficult.

The Calibrated Small-caliber-tip Transparent (CAST) hood, manufactured by TOP Co. (Fig. 4.6) [20], is a specialized hood with a narrow, transparent tip and calibration markings. When the hood is pressed against the stricture, the guidewire emerging from the working channel contacts the inner surface of the hood and is directed to the center of the screen, facilitating passage through the stricture. Furthermore, by pressing the hood against the stricture and observing the appearance of a white circular ring, the calibration markings on the hood can be used to measure the inner diameter of the stricture (Fig. 4.7). The CAST hood also simplifies advancing the endoscope beyond the stricture after EBD, allowing sequential EBD of multiple strictures during a single procedure.

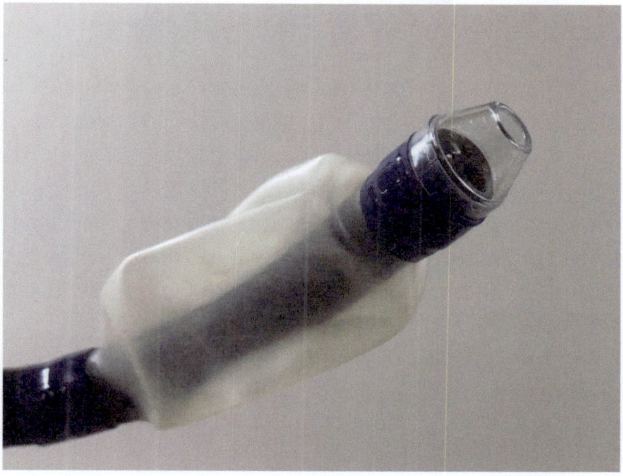

Fig. 4.6 CAST hood

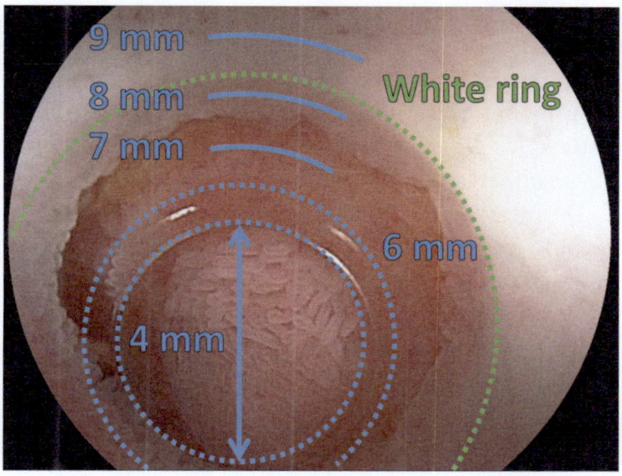

Fig. 4.7 Endoscopic image with the CAST hood

4.8.7 Selection of Equipment

For dilation, balloon catheters with hemispherical (barrel-shaped) ends are preferred. At our institution, we use the CRE Pro GI Wire-Guided Balloon Dilator (Boston Scientific, No. 5881–5883), which is designed for lower gastrointestinal tract use and offers practical size options. However, the guidewire preloaded in the dilator is often too stiff for small intestinal procedures. Instead, a 0.035-inch diameter guidewire, commonly used in biliary interventions, is utilized to ensure smoother and safer navigation during the procedure.

4.8.8 Minimal Water Exchange Method

During endoscopy, insufflation causes bowel distension, which can reduce insertion efficiency. Residual gas in the intestine can also hinder the shortening maneuvers of BAE. Additionally, EBD can cause minor vascular disruption, posing risks of portal venous gas or gas embolism [21]. Therefore, the use of carbon dioxide insufflation is essential, and a no-insufflation, water-assisted approach is ideal. A prospective randomized trial demonstrated that the water exchange method, replacing intestinal gas and fluid with water, improves the completion rate of total enteroscopy during BAE [22].

At our institution, we employ the minimal water exchange method [23], which replaces intestinal fluid and residual gas with the smallest possible volume of water. Filling the CAST hood with a small amount of water provides sufficient visibility. Water is introduced via the endoscope's water button rather than the working channel. Using the working channel for water infusion mixes the pathways for suction and irrigation, pushing back intestinal fluid and making it harder to maintain a clear view. Alternatively, water can be injected through the water-jet channel with a pump, but care must be taken to avoid overfilling. Eliminating all residual gas prevents foam formation, allowing for a consistently clear view. Underwater conditions also reduce glare (halation) and improve the transparency of the CAST hood, creating an effect similar to the dome of a capsule endoscope.

During selective contrast studies, the absence of residual gas allows the contrast agent to diffuse smoothly through the intestinal fluid. This results in seamless imaging of the small intestine, even in the presence of bowel angulation, deformation, or strictures. When using the scope's water button, just blocking the central hole of the button results in insufflation. To avoid this, the edge of the button should be pressed fast and strongly. By employing these techniques, our institution performs BAE entirely in an underwater, no-insufflation state from the time the scope passes the anus or the pylorus to the completion of the treatment procedure.

4.8.9 Target Dilation Diameter

Selecting an appropriate dilation diameter is crucial to achieve sufficient therapeutic effect while avoiding the risk of perforation. The target diameter must strike a balance, stopping just short of excessive expansion. When in doubt, opting for a smaller dilation diameter is safer. Using the CAST hood, the inner diameter of the stricture is measured to guide the selection of the dilation balloon catheter. For strictures with an inner diameter of 4 mm or less, the target dilation diameter is 8–10 mm. For strictures with an inner diameter of 5–7 mm, the target dilation diameter is 10–12 mm. For strictures with an inner diameter of 8 mm or more, the target dilation diameter is 12–15 mm. The choice of dilation diameter should be based on a comprehensive assessment, considering factors such as the measured stricture diameter, stricture length, the presence of ulcers, the maximum dilation diameter achieved during the previous EBD session, and the total number of strictures requiring treatment.

4.8.10 Insertion of the Dilation Balloon Catheter

As previously mentioned, the standard guidewire preloaded in the balloon catheter should not be used. Instead, a thinner and more flexible 0.035-inch guidewire should be threaded to the tip of the dilation balloon catheter in advance. Once the dilation balloon catheter is inserted, it should remain in place until all strictures requiring EBD have been treated. To facilitate this, ensure that the BioShield® irrigator is attached beforehand. Even with a scope featuring a 3.2-mm working channel, once the balloon catheter has been expanded, re-insertion can encounter significant resistance. To improve maneuverability, 0.5–1 ml of olive oil can be injected into the working channel immediately before inserting the balloon catheter. However, excessive use of olive oil should be avoided, as it may adhere to the endoscope lens and impair visibility.

4.8.11 Adjusting Intestinal Shape and Balloon Position

When the dilation balloon is inflated, it becomes a rigid rod approximately 5 cm long. If the intestinal tract is angulated at the site of the stricture, this rigidity may create excessive pressure on the intestinal wall proximal or distal to the stricture, increasing the risk of perforation. To prevent this, the intestinal shape should be adjusted before balloon inflation. In DBE, the intestinal shape can be corrected by grasping the intestine with the scope-tip balloon and manipulating the endoscope to straighten the affected segment.

The intestinal shape, proximal dilation, and stricture length can be evaluated using selective contrast imaging with a 2× diluted water-soluble contrast agent. However, when performing EBD on multiple strictures consecutively, contrast imaging can be omitted or limited to minimal injections to streamline the procedure. If the relationship between the dilation balloon catheter and the stricture needs to be reassessed after catheter insertion, additional contrast medium can be injected through the BioShield® irrigator to confirm the positioning. This ensures accurate and safe dilation while minimizing risks associated with improper catheter alignment.

4.8.12 Gradual Balloon Dilation

Dilation with the balloon should be performed gradually, starting from the smallest diameter and increasing step by step. The initial dilation phase requires particular caution, with the balloon being slowly inflated to the specified pressure. At our institution, the balloon is inflated and held for 1 min in each dilation step. After each step, the condition of the stricture, the presence of bleeding, and the patient's pain level are assessed to determine whether to proceed to the next diameter. If any concerns arise, further dilation is avoided, as intestinal perforation would negate the procedure's benefits. This careful, incremental approach ensures the safety and the efficacy of the dilation process while minimizing the risk of complications.

4.8.13 Scope Passage After EBD

Dilation of the stricture to 12 mm typically allows passage of the endoscope, while dilation to 13.5 mm is often sufficient for the overtube to pass. However, depending on the shape and angulation of the intestine, passage may still be difficult. In such cases, leaving the dilation balloon catheter or guidewire in place at the stricture site can facilitate passage. If the mucosa is significantly torn, exposing the muscular layer, attempts to pass the scope should be avoided. This is especially critical for overtube passage, as it involves blind manipulation, which carries higher risks. The decision to pass the scope or overtube should be carefully weighed, considering both the necessity of the procedure and the associated risks. Safety should always take precedence in these situations.

4.8.14 Sequential EBD for Multiple Strictures

When performing EBD for multiple strictures, the CAST hood facilitates the endoscope's passage beyond dilated strictures. If strictures are distributed over a wide area, deep insertion of the endoscope and the overtube may be required. Strictures that permit endoscope passage but obstruct overtube passage should be dilated to 13.5 mm during insertion. Dilation beyond this, such as 15 mm, may cause the dilation balloon to elongate, making it difficult to retract through the working channel. Thus, dilation should be limited to 13.5 mm in these cases.

For multiple strictures, completely removing and reinserting the dilation balloon catheter after each EBD would be highly labor-intensive. Instead, the catheter can be retracted into the working channel after each dilation, avoiding the need for complete removal. As noted earlier, if multiple strictures are widespread and cannot all be addressed via a single insertion route, EBD should be attempted through both oral and anal routes to ensure comprehensive treatment. This bidirectional approach increases the likelihood of treating all strictures effectively while minimizing procedural challenges.

4.8.15 Post-EBD Management and Medication

The patient's abdominal symptoms are assessed in the morning after the procedure. If no symptoms are present, oral intake is gradually resumed, starting with elemental diets or liquid foods. At our institution, oral fluoroquinolone antibiotics are administered for 5 days starting on the day of the procedure to address potential bacterial translocation caused by temporary mucosal barrier disruption. To minimize post-EBD edema and fibrosis, a tapering course of oral prednisolone is prescribed: 30 mg/day for 2 days, 20 mg/day for the next 2 days, and 10 mg/day for the final 2 days, resulting in a total treatment duration of 6 days. This regimen helps reduce complications and promotes a smoother recovery following EBD.

4.8.16 Adverse Events of EBD

At our institution, among the 720 EBD procedures performed for Crohn's disease-associated small intestinal strictures using DBE up to the end of August 2019, significant bleeding with a hemoglobin drop of ≥2 g/dL occurred in five cases (0.7%). Of these, two required blood transfusions or endoscopic hemostasis. Perforation occurred in four cases (0.6%), all of which necessitated emergency surgery. In addition to adverse events directly related to the EBD procedure, the potential for complications arising from BAE insertion itself must also be considered in Crohn's disease. The disease often involves transmural inflammation of the intestinal wall, leading to the formation of deep ulcers. Even after remission induction, while these ulcers may appear healed, the muscular layer may not have regained sufficient strength. Furthermore, inflammation often extends to the mesentery, causing fibrosis and shortening (Fig. 4.8).

During endoscope insertion, the forces exerted on the mesenteric attachment points are normally distributed evenly in a smooth arc if the mesentery retains its original length. However, in areas where the mesentery is fibrotic and shortened, forces are concentrated, often coinciding with regions of insufficient muscular

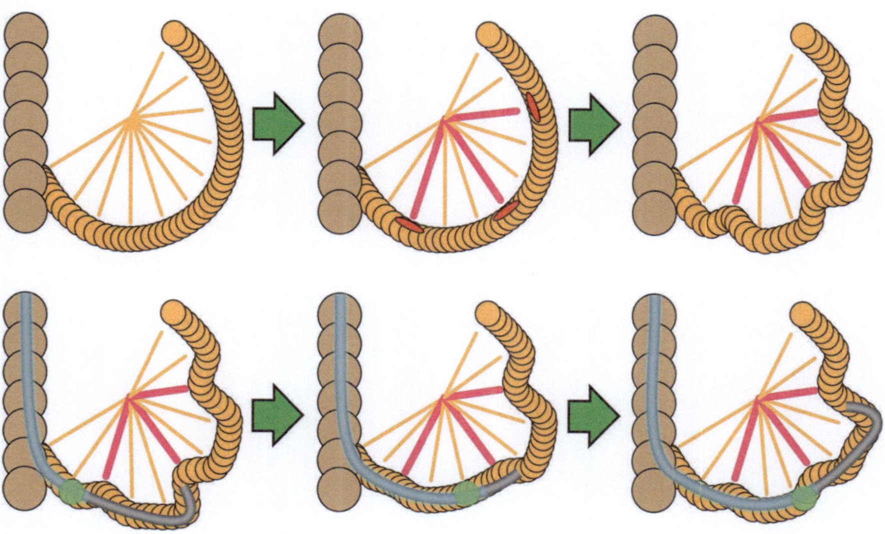

Fig. 4.8 Difficulty of scope insertion due to a scarred and shortened mesentery

strength, increasing the risk of perforation (Fig. 4.9). Such perforations typically occur in areas the endoscope has already passed, making them difficult to detect solely through the endoscopic view. The appearance of blood-tinged intestinal fluid in the overtube or endoscopic field during the procedure should be regarded as a warning sign of potential perforation.

If symptoms suggestive of perforation, such as severe abdominal pain, arise after BAE, an abdominal CT scan should be performed to confirm its presence. If perforation is detected during the procedure, endoscopic closure using clips may be attempted, although success is often limited. If closure is not feasible, it is crucial to avoid reliance on conservative management and proceed with surgical treatment at an appropriate time to ensure patient safety.

4.8.17 Follow-Up After EBD

If deep remission is maintained after EBD, repeated procedures often result in improvements in both the number and diameter of strictures. Conversely, failure to maintain deep remission not only worsens the number and diameter of strictures [24], but also exacerbates bowel deformation and mesenteric shortening, making it increasingly difficult to access strictures. When signs of inflammation are detected, it is crucial to optimize medical therapy proactively.

For residual strictures, dietary restrictions should be continued, and repeat EBD should be performed 2–6 months later. Once all strictures have been dilated to at least 12 mm, follow-up BAE can be performed 6–12 months later to dilate the strictures further to 15 mm. Subsequently, BAE should be conducted annually for disease evaluation, with EBD performed as needed.

If rapid re-stricturing occurs, necessitating EBD at intervals of less than 6 months, surgical treatment should be considered. Prior to surgery, both oral and anal

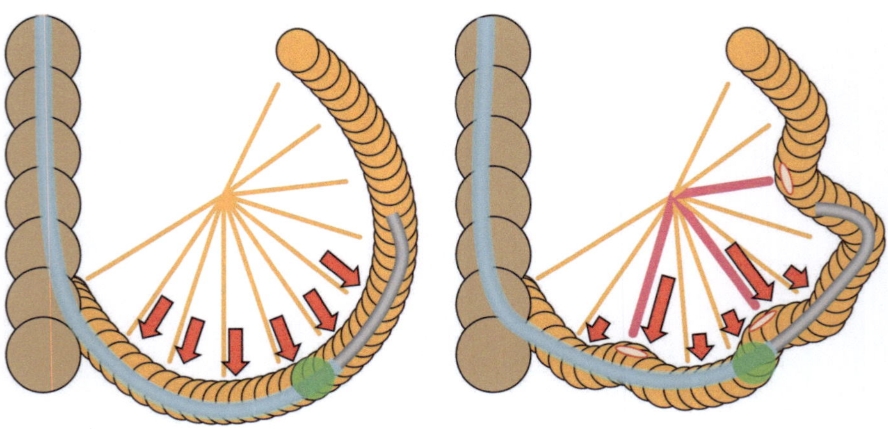

Fig. 4.9 Excessive forces generated in an already pathological small bowel by a scarred and shortened mesentery

routes of BAE should be used to assess the remaining length of the small intestine and mark critical areas with tattooing.

When partial small bowel resection is performed, functional end-to-end anastomosis can result in a high frequency of anastomotic strictures, which also complicates endoscopic passage through the anastomosis in future endoscopic procedures. In contrast, the Kono-S anastomosis has a lower incidence of anastomotic strictures and facilitates easier endoscopic insertion across the anastomotic site [25, 26].

4.9 Summary

Balloon-assisted endoscopy (BAE) has made it possible to perform endoscopic interventions even in the deep small intestine. However, to ensure safe and effective procedures, a thorough understanding of the anatomical characteristics of the small intestine is essential.

References

1. Yano T, Nemoto D, Ono K, et al. Gel immersion endoscopy: a novel method to secure the visual field during endoscopy in bleeding patients (with videos). Gastrointest Endosc. 2016;83:809–11.
2. Yano K, Yano T, Nagayama M, et al. Hemostasis of an actively bleeding lesion at the ileocecal valve by low-pressure endoscopy using the gel immersion technique. VideoGIE. 2021;6:184–6.
3. Yano T, Yamamoto H, Sunada K, et al. Endoscopic classification of vascular lesions of the small intestine (with videos). Gastrointest Endosc. 2008;67:169–72.
4. Owada J, Kihara A, Yano T. Novel cold snare technique with clipping for duodenal angioectasia. Dig Endosc. 2024;36:499–501.
5. Miura Y, Shinozaki S, Hayashi Y, et al. Duodenal endoscopic submucosal dissection is feasible using the pocket-creation method. Endoscopy. 2017;49:8–14.
6. Oguro K, Sakamoto H, Yano T, et al. Endoscopic treatment of intussusception due to small intestine polyps in patients with Peutz-Jeghers syndrome. Endosc Int Open. 2022;10:E1583–8.
7. Matsumoto T, Esaki M, Yanaru-Fujisawa R, et al. Small-intestinal involvement in familial adenomatous polyposis: evaluation by double-balloon endoscopy and intraoperative enteroscopy. Gastrointest Endosc. 2008;68:911–9.
8. van Leerdam ME, Roos VH, van Hooft JE, et al. Endoscopic management of polyposis syndromes: European Society of Gastrointestinal Endoscopy (ESGE) guideline. Endoscopy. 2019;51:877–95.
9. Iida M, Sakamoto H, Miura Y, et al. Jejunal endoscopic submucosal dissection is feasible using the pocket-creation method and balloon-assisted endoscopy. Endoscopy. 2018;50:931–2.
10. Sekiya M, Sakamoto H, Yano T, et al. Double-balloon endoscopy facilitates efficient endoscopic resection of duodenal and jejunal polyps in patients with familial adenomatous polyposis. Endoscopy. 2020; https://doi.org/10.1055/a-1189-9550.
11. Takeuchi Y, Hamada K, Nakahira H, et al. Efficacy and safety of intensive downstaging polypectomy (IDP) for multiple duodenal adenomas in patients with familial adenomatous polyposis: a prospective cohort study. Endoscopy. 2023;55:515–23.
12. Iwata K, Kato M, Sasaki M, et al. Intensive endoscopic resection strategy for multiple duodenal polyposis associated with familial adenomatous polyposis. J Gastroenterol Hepatol. 2023;38:1592–7.

13. Dofuku M, Yano T, Yokoyama K, et al. Management of pediatric Peutz-Jeghers syndrome: highlighting the efficacy and safety of endoscopic ischemic polypectomy. J Pediatr Gastroenterol Nutr. 2025; https://doi.org/10.1002/jpn3.12458.
14. Khurelbaatar T, Sakamoto H, Yano T, et al. Endoscopic ischemic polypectomy for small-intestinal polyps in patients with Peutz-Jeghers syndrome. Endoscopy. 2020; https://doi.org/10.1055/a-1276-6452.
15. Yano T, Shinozaki S, Yamamoto H. Crossed-clip strangulation for the management of small intestinal polyps in patients with Peutz-Jeghers syndrome. Dig Endosc. 2018;30:677.
16. Takakura K, Kato T, Arihiro S, et al. Selective ligation using a detachable snare for small-intestinal polyps in patients with Peutz-Jeghers syndrome. Endoscopy. 2011;43(Suppl 2):E264–5.
17. Tamaru T, Oguro K, Yano T, et al. Clip-and-pull method: re-strangulation of a sizable small-bowel polyp for endoscopic ischemic polypectomy. Endoscopy. 2024;56:E424–5.
18. Funayama Y, Oguro K, Sakamoto H, et al. Repeat bidirectional double-balloon enteroscopy 1 year later may be proper in Peutz-Jeghers patients with difficult-to-reach polyps. Endosc Int Open. 2023;11:E1110–5.
19. Ono Y, Oguro K, Yano T, et al. Ischemic polypectomy using a diagnostic-type double-balloon endoscope with a modified detachable snare. Endoscopy. 2023;55:E294–6.
20. Hayashi Y, Yamamoto H, Yano T, et al. A calibrated, small-caliber tip, transparent hood to aid endoscopic balloon dilation of intestinal strictures in Crohn's disease: successful use of prototype. Endoscopy. 2013;45(Suppl 2):E373–4.
21. Takahashi F, Tominaga K, Hiraishi H. Hepatic portal venous gas caused by endoscopic balloon dilatation for Crohn's stenosis. Clin Gastroenterol Hepatol. 2016;14:A23–a24.
22. Liu S, Dong T, Shi Y, et al. Water exchange-assisted versus carbon dioxide-insufflated single-balloon enteroscopy: a randomized controlled trial. Endoscopy. 2022;54:281–9.
23. Yeh JH, Chien HY. Minimal water exchange colonoscopy. VideoGIE. 2019;4:56–7.
24. Dashnyam U, Nagayama M, Yano T, et al. Maintenance of complete mucosal healing is associated with avoiding restenosis after endoscopic balloon dilation of Crohn's disease-related small intestinal strictures. DEN Open. 2023;3:e239.
25. Kono T, Ashida T, Ebisawa Y, et al. A new antimesenteric functional end-to-end handsewn anastomosis: surgical prevention of anastomotic recurrence in Crohn's disease. Dis Colon Rectum. 2011;54:586–92.
26. Ng CH, Chin YH, Lin SY, et al. Kono-S anastomosis for Crohn's disease: a systemic review, meta-analysis, and meta-regression. Surg Today. 2021;51:493–501.

Application of Balloon-Assisted Enteroscopy in Special Situations

5

Dong-Hoon Yang and Eun Ran Kim

5.1 Altered Anatomical Structures

5.1.1 Introduction

Balloon-assisted enteroscopy (BAE) has enabled endoscopic procedures in patients with postoperative anatomical alterations, inaccessible with conventional endoscopy. In clinical practice, the most common scenario for applying BAE in patients with surgically altered anatomy is to perform endoscopic retrograde cholangiopancreatography (ERCP) in patients with lesions in the afferent loop of Roux-en-Y anastomosis. In patients who have undergone Billroth II subtotal gastrectomy (Fig. 5.1) or various surgeries involving Roux-en-Y anastomosis (Table 5.1, Fig. 5.2), endoscopic access to the afferent loop is limited or impossible without BAE. However, BAE allows access to such sites and enables diagnostic and therapeutic interventions for gastrointestinal bleeding, choledocholithiasis, and other pancreaticobiliary problems. The basic insertion principles of BAE are similar to those used in patients with normal anatomy. However, in patients with surgically altered anatomy, endoscopists should be familiar with the anatomical changes before performing BAE. Therefore, the endoscopist should acquire sufficient pre-procedural information about the relevant surgery by reviewing surgical records and consulting with the surgeon to understand the individual postoperative anatomy of each patient. If BAE is performed not for simple hemostasis but for ERCP, collaboration and discussion with a pancreatobiliary endoscopist are essential for procedural planning.

D.-H. Yang (✉)
University of Ulsan College of Medicine, Seoul, South Korea
e-mail: dhyang@amc.seoul.kr

E. R. Kim
Sungkyunkwan University School of Medicine, Seoul, South Korea
e-mail: er.kim@samsung.com

J.-J. Park et al. (eds.), *Balloon-Assisted Enteroscopy*,
https://doi.org/10.1007/978-981-95-2445-7_5

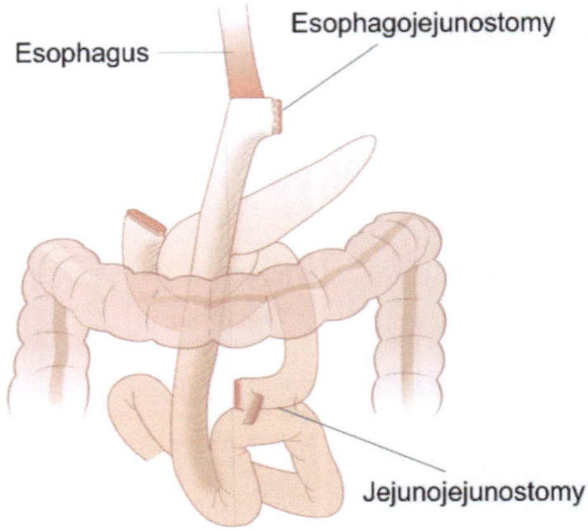

Fig. 5.1 Anatomical alteration after Billroth II subtotal gastrectomy

Table 5.1 Various operations including Roux-en-Y anastomosis

Type of operation	Biliary drainage site
Short-limb roux-en-Y (<50 cm)	
Whipple resection with roux-en-Y hepaico and pancreaticojejunostomy	Bilioenteric anastomosis
Biliary diversion with roux-en-Y hepaico and pancreaticojejunostomy	Bilioenteric anastomosis
Total gastrectomy with roux-en-Y esophagojejunostomy	Intact papilla
Long-limb roux-en-Y (>100 cm)	
Scopinaro roux-en-Y biliopancreatic diversion	Intact papilla
Roux-en-Y gastric bypass	Intact papilla

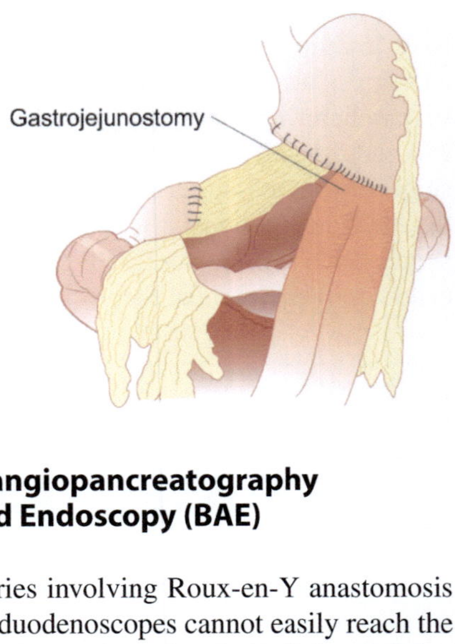

Fig. 5.2 Altered anatomy after Billroth II subtotal gastrectomy

5.1.2 Endoscopic Retrograde Cholangiopancreatography (ERCP) Using Balloon-Assisted Endoscopy (BAE)

Patients who have undergone various surgeries involving Roux-en-Y anastomosis or Billroth II operation, where conventional duodenoscopes cannot easily reach the duodenal papilla, are the primary candidates for ERCP using BAE. It is crucial to thoroughly review the patient's surgical records and, if possible, consult the operating surgeon to obtain detailed information about the postoperative anatomy. Additionally, pre-procedural imaging studies such as abdominal computed tomography (CT), magnetic resonance imaging (MRI), or small bowel follow-through can provide information about the anatomical alterations.

The basic insertion techniques of BAE to perform ERCP are similar to those used in patients with normal anatomy. However, postoperative intraabdominal adhesions can restrict the mobility of the small intestine, making BAE insertion more challenging. In cases where resistance is encountered, forceful advancement of the endoscope should be avoided. Instead, fluoroscopic guidance can help assess loop formation and direction. Minimizing air insufflation and utilizing positional changes or abdominal compression can facilitate scope advancement.

When the anastomosis is not identified during insertion, continued advancement may lead the enteroscope in the wrong direction (e.g., efferent loop instead of afferent loop). If the enteroscope has advanced approximately 120–140 cm and the tip is observed in the central abdomen or pelvis on fluoroscopy, this often indicates that the scope has entered the efferent loop. In that situation, the enteroscope should be slowly withdrawn to find the anastomosis. If the anastomosis or suture clips are not directly visible, clues such as the disappearance of Kerckring's folds, reverse peristalsis, or the presence of bile are useful to identify the anastomosis. A sudden widening of the lumen may also indicate proximity to the anastomosis, and thus this area should be carefully examined to figure out surgical scars or dual lumens (Table 5.2, Fig. 5.3) [1].

To enter the afferent loop after identifying the jejuno-jejunostomy, the endoscope should be advanced into the laterally bifurcated lumen or into the lumen containing bile or yellowish foam. The final path of the afferent loop leads toward the remaining duodenum or biliary-enteric anastomosis (e.g., hepaticojejunostomy or choledochojejunostomy). Therefore, the tip of the endoscope will eventually be directed toward the patient's right upper abdomen, forming an angle with the efferent loop at the anastomosis. To advance deeper into the afferent loop, the enteroscope should be inserted 15–20 cm beyond the anastomosis. After fixing the tip of endoscope at this position, the overtube should be advanced. Once the overtube is advanced to the maximal depth near the tip of the enteroscope, the overtube balloon is inflated to keep its position, allowing further advancement of the enteroscope into the afferent loop.

Table 5.2 Balloon-assisted enteroscopy (BAE) findings useful to identify anastomosis site or afferent loop in patients with surgically altered anatomy

1. Anastomotic scarring and the presence of suture clips allow direct observation of the anastomotic site
2. Loss of small bowel transverse folds (Kerkring's folds) suggests the presence of an anastomosis
3. Sudden widening of the lumen during BAE insertion suggests a nearby anastomosis
4. Afferent loop indicated by bile staining or peristalsis opposite to insertion

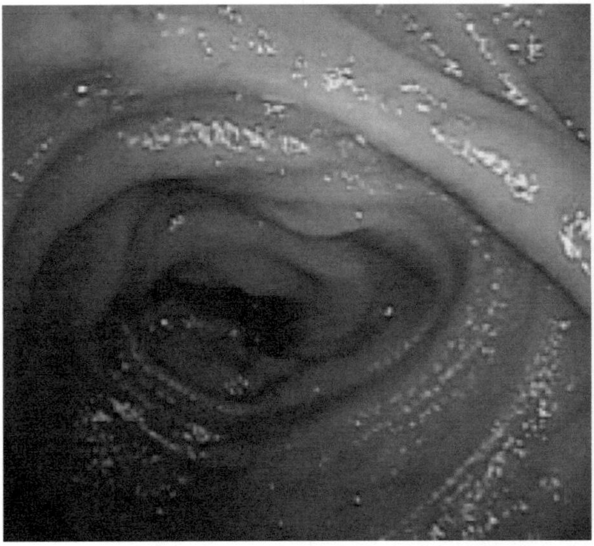

Fig. 5.3 Endoscopic finding of jejunojejunostomyThe anastomotic scar is observed at the top of the endoscopic image and the endoscope can be advanced into the afferent loop through the 1 o'clock side

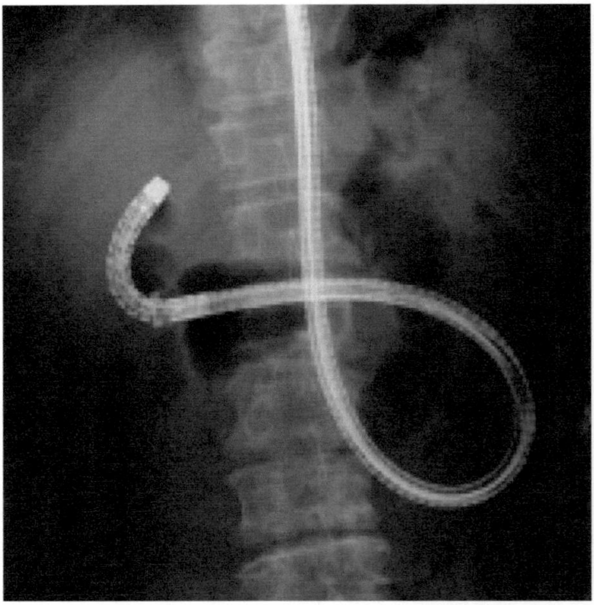

Fig. 5.4 Fluoroscopic image of the balloon-assisted enteroscope inserted into the afferent loop The enteroscope is positioned in a figure of eight with the tip of the enteroscope directed toward the hepatic shadow

When fluoroscopy reveals the enteroscope tip near the hepatic shadow or when the scope appears coiled in a spiral or figure-eight pattern (Fig. 5.4), this indicates deep insertion into the afferent loop. Then, the biliary-enteric anastomosis, duodenal stump, or major papilla should be identified. The location of these landmarks varies in patients with surgically altered anatomy, but they are generally observed in the left or lower-left portion of the endoscopic view. Once the biliary-enteric

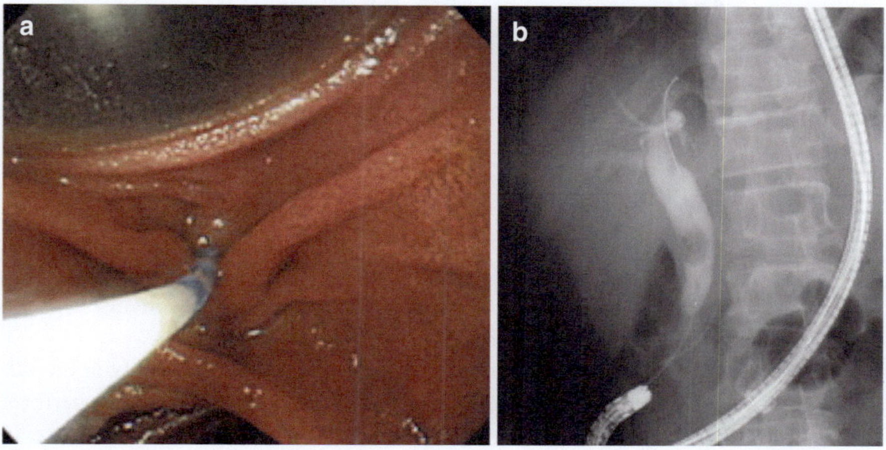

Fig. 5.5 ERCP performed with single-balloon enteroscopy in a patient who underwent total gastrectomy and Roux-en-Y anastomosis. (**a**) The duodenal papilla was approached with a single-balloon enteroscope and the overtube was retained and replaced with a gastroscope. The catheter is inserted into the papilla, and the overtube balloon is observed at 12 o'clock. (**b**) The cholangiogram shows an opacification due to a common bile duct stone, which was removed after mechanical lithotripsy

anastomosis or duodenal papilla is located, a guidewire can be introduced to access the bile duct, followed by the necessary diagnostic or therapeutic interventions.

Due to the 200-cm working length of the enteroscope, the range of accessories available for ERCP through the small bowel enteroscope is limited (Fig. 5.5). However, the short-type BAEs (short-type double-balloon enteroscopy [DBE]: EI-580BT, length of enteroscope: 155 cm, working channel diameter: 3.2 mm; short-type single-balloon enteroscopy [SBE]: SIF-H290S; length of enteroscope: 152 cm, working channel diameter: 3.2 mm) allow the use of standard ERCP accessories.

5.1.3 Clinical Outcomes of BAE-Assisted ERCP

BAE-assisted ERCP was first introduced to resolve biliary problems in patients who underwent Roux-en-Y anastomosis using a DBE. Subsequently, BAE-assisted ERCP has been reported not only with DBE but also with SBE and short-type BAE. The majority of BAE-assisted ERCPs are performed to treat biliary problems, and the main indications are biliary-enteric anastomotic stricture or common bile duct stones in patients who have undergone a Roux-en-Y anastomosis.

A meta-analysis of 24 studies including 1523 patients, published between 2001 and 2017, reported an overall diagnostic success rate of 94% and a procedural success rate of 93% for ERCP using DBE. Notably, there was no significant difference in diagnostic and procedural success rates according to the length of the DBE used [2]. In addition, the incidence of procedure-related complications was 4%, including pancreatitis, perforation, and cholangitis. With the exception of one patient who underwent emergency laparotomy for perforation, all patients were managed conservatively and there were no complication-related deaths [2]. According to a recent meta-analysis including 21 studies and 1227 cases of SBE-assisted ERCP, the success rate of SBE-assisted ERCP was 76% and the complication rate was 6.6% [3]. While the success rate with SBE appears somewhat lower compared to DBE, the heterogeneity of the studies included in both meta-analyses limits direct comparison. A retrospective study that directly compared the results of DBE- and SBE-assisted ERCP in patients undergoing Roux-en-Y gastric bypass showed that the success rates of ERCP were 73% and 75%, respectively, with no difference depending on the type of BAE [4].

Bowel perforation is the most serious complication, occurring mainly at the biliary-enteric anastomosis or near the duodenal papilla. It is recommended to perform BAE at least 2 weeks after Roux-en-Y anastomosis to avoid anastomotic injury. In most cases where BAE is performed to evaluate pancreaticobiliary problems rather than for bleeding, several months or years have passed since the surgery, so the risk of anastomotic site injury is generally low. However, most ERCP procedures are performed at or near to the blind end of the afferent loop after stabilizing the scope position by the inflated overtube balloon. So, excessive or prolonged gas insufflation in that situation can rapidly increase the intraluminal pressure of the blind loop, potentially causing air leakage from the biliary-enteric anastomosis and papillary sphincterotomy into the peritoneal or retroperitoneal cavity. In addition to perforation, bleeding, cholangitis, or pancreatitis may occur after ERCP, though these are usually mild and resolve with conservative treatment. Mucosal injury and subsequent bleeding in the stomach or afferent loop due to mechanical pressure from BAE have also been reported and can be managed with conservative treatment.

5.1.4 Conclusion

In order to perform an effective enteroscopic procedure in patients with surgically altered anatomy, the endoscopist should be familiar with and have knowledge of both the normal and surgically altered anatomy of the gastrointestinal tract. BAE-assisted ERCP is useful in resolving pancreaticobiliary problems in patients with surgically altered anatomy. For BAE-assisted ERCP to be successful, there must be a collaborative effort between the BAE endoscopist, the surgeon, and the ERCP endoscopist.

5.2 Difficult Colonoscopy Insertion

5.2.1 Introduction

Colonoscopy is widely regarded as the most effective approach for colorectal cancer prevention through the detection and removal of colon polyps. Achieving cecal intubation is a key quality indicator for the procedure. However, studies show that even skilled endoscopists fail to reach the cecum in about 10% of cases. According to the American Society for Gastrointestinal Endoscopy guidelines, a cecal intubation rate exceeding 90% is recommended for all colonoscopies, with a rate over 95% for screening colonoscopies in healthy adults as a standard of quality [5].

Factors that can hinder cecal intubation include prior abdominal surgery, a colon that is prone to loop formation, a rigid or sharply angled colon, diverticular disease, low body mass index, poor bowel preparation, and limited operator skill [6, 7].

Studies indicate that reattempting the procedure in such cases achieves successful cecal intubation in 94–98% of instances [7, 8]. Ensuring adequate sedation and minimizing loop formation with an adult colonoscope can facilitate reaching the cecum. For cases involving a fixed or angled colon, a pediatric colonoscope or gastroscope may be effective, while a variable-stiffness colonoscope can be beneficial for a lengthy, loop-prone colon. Despite these approaches, cecal intubation remains unattainable in 1–3% of cases due to the technical complexity and time involved.

5.2.2 Alternative Examinations for Patients with Difficult Cecal Intubation

Various imaging methods may be used as alternatives for cases of incomplete colonoscopy. Double-contrast barium enema was once used to detect colorectal cancer in such patients; however, it missed 20% of proximal colon cancers and detected only 50% of polyps. Its diagnostic rate was significantly lower than that of reattempting colonoscopy (34.3% vs. 3.6%, $p < 0.0001$), and it is no longer recommended as an alternative for incomplete colonoscopy [7, 9].

Computed tomography (CT) or magnetic resonance (MR) colonography are viable alternatives, with CT colonography having about 90% sensitivity for polyps over 10 mm in asymptomatic patients, making it useful for cases of incomplete colonoscopy. MR colonography, although free from radiation exposure, is less standardized and less widely available than CT colonography.

The European Society of Gastrointestinal Endoscopy (ESGE) advises using CT colonography as an alternative test for patients with symptoms of colorectal cancer when conventional colonoscopy is not possible, as it offers similar sensitivity.

5.2.3 Device-Assisted Small Bowel Endoscopy for Patients with Difficult Cecal Intubation

5.2.3.1 Device-Assisted Small Bowel Enteroscopy

Device-assisted small bowel enteroscopy, designed for deep access into the small bowel, includes techniques such as balloon-assisted small bowel enteroscopy. This method involves double-balloon or single-balloon enteroscope, where the balloons are attached to both the overtube and endoscope or only to the overtube, respectively. Balloon-assisted enteroscopy stabilizes the colon using an overtube balloon, reducing loop formation during insertion of the enteroscope and overtube. This method is effective for patients with lengthy or loop-prone colons, as it prevents loops from forming and allows reentry by shortening existing loops. For angulated or fixed colon segments, the overtube balloon stabilizes the fixed area, helping the endoscope maneuver through narrow, angled sections to achieve cecal intubation.

In cases of incomplete colonoscopy, the cecal intubation rate with double-balloon enteroscope ranges from 88% to 100%, with intubation times between 15 and 48 min. For single-balloon enteroscope, cecal intubation rates are between 93% and 100%, with insertion times of 12–40 min [7].

In a recent study of 122 patients with incomplete colonoscopy, balloon-assisted small bowel enteroscopy achieved a cecal intubation rate of 92.6%, with failure rates of 8.3% (1 of 12) for single-balloon and 7.3% (8 of 110) for double-balloon enteroscopy. Success rates varied based on the cause of the initial failure: 84.6% in patients with a history of abdominal surgery, 96.3% in those with abdominal discomfort, and 90.7% in those with angulation or diverticular disease, highlighting the effectiveness of balloon-assisted enteroscopy in challenging cases [10]. A comparison between single-balloon and double-balloon enteroscopy showed cecal intubation rates of 100% (26 of 26) and 93% (25 of 27), with no significant difference between the two methods [11].

Balloon-assisted enteroscopy has also shown effectiveness when compared to reattempted colonoscopy. In a study involving 30 patients who underwent both reattempted colonoscopy and single-balloon enteroscopy, cecal intubation rates were 50% for reattempted colonoscopy and 93% for single-balloon enteroscopy. Notably, single-balloon enteroscopy successfully achieved cecal intubation in all patients where reattempted colonoscopy had failed [12].

However, balloon-assisted enteroscopy has limitations, such as the high cost of the overtube, handling difficulties, and radiation exposure. To address these issues, using a balloon only at the endoscope tip, without an overtube, has been shown to achieve cecal intubation rates of 91–93.4%. This method is especially useful for patients with angulated and fixed colon segments or diverticular disease, where enteroscopic access is more challenging [13].

Another type of device-assisted enteroscopy uses a spiral overtube instead of a balloon. In a study of 24 patients with incomplete colonoscopy, the spiral overtube achieved a cecal intubation rate of 92% (22 of 24). However, research on spiral overtubes is limited, and they are not yet commercially available [14].

5.2.3.2 New Forms of Device-Assisted Enteroscopy

Recently, new device-assisted enteroscopes have been developed to assist with cecal intubation. One such device is the NaviAid G-EYE® (Smart Medical Systems Ltd., Ra'anana, Israel), which features a balloon on the bending section of the colonoscope to aid in cecal intubation. Another innovation involves inserting a catheter with an integrated balloon into the biopsy channel of the colonoscope, known as the NaviAid™ Advancing Balloon for Colonoscopy (NaviAid ABC, Smart Medical Systems).

The NaviAid™ AB (Advancing Balloon) is a catheter designed to fit into the biopsy channel of a colonoscope. During cecal intubation, the balloon at the catheter's tip is inflated to stabilize it against the colon wall, allowing the colonoscope to advance along the catheter and reducing loop formation. It has been reported that cecal intubation was successfully achieved in all nine patients who underwent incomplete colonoscopy using this device.

The NaviAid G-EYE® was theoretically expected to be helpful for patients with incomplete colonoscopy. However, there is currently no research demonstrating its effectiveness in this specific group of patients.

Both auxiliary endoscopic devices have limited research regarding their use in patients with incomplete colonoscopy [7, 15].

References

1. Moreels TG. Altered anatomy: enteroscopy and ERCP procedure. Best Pract Res Clin Gastroenterol. 2012;26:347–57.
2. Anvari S, Lee Y, Patro N, et al. Double-balloon enteroscopy for diagnostic and therapeutic ERCP in patients with surgically altered gastrointestinal anatomy: a systematic review and meta-analysis. Surg Endosc. 2020;
3. Tanisaka Y, Ryozawa S, Mizuide M, et al. Status of single-balloon enteroscopy-assisted ERCP in patients with surgically altered anatomy: a systematic review and meta-analysis on biliary interventions. Dig Endosc. 2020;
4. De Koning M, Moreels TG. Comparison of double-balloon and single-balloon enteroscope for therapeutic endoscopic retrograde cholangiography after roux-en-Y small bowel surgery. BMC Gastroenterol. 2016;16:98.
5. Rex DK, Schoenfeld PS, Cohen J, et al. Quality indicators for colonoscopy. Gastrointest Endosc. 2015;81:31–53.
6. Kaltenbach T, Soetikno R, Friedland S. Use of a double balloon enteroscope facilitates caecal intubation after incomplete colonoscopy with a standard colonoscope. Dig Liver Dis. 2006;38:921–5.
7. Villa NA, Pannala R, Pasha SF, et al. Alternatives to incomplete colonoscopy. Curr Gastroenterol Rep. 2015;17:43.
8. Rex DK, Chen SC, Overhiser AJ. Colonoscopy technique in consecutive patients referred for prior incomplete colonoscopy. Clin Gastroenterol Hepatol. 2007;5:879–83.
9. Spada C, Hassan C, Bellini D, et al. Imaging alternatives to colonoscopy: CT colonography and colon capsule. European Society of Gastrointestinal Endoscopy (ESGE) and European Society of Gastrointestinal and Abdominal Radiology (ESGAR) guideline – update 2020. Eur Radiol. 2021;31:2967–82.
10. Robertson AR, Koulaouzidis A, Yung DE, et al. Balloon-assisted colonoscopy after incomplete conventional colonoscopy-experience from two European centres with a comprehensive review of the miterature. J Clin Med. 2020;9:2981.
11. Dzeletovic I, Harrison ME, Pasha SF, et al. Comparison of single- versus double-balloon assisted-colonoscopy for colon examination after previous incomplete standard colonoscopy. Dig Dis Sci. 2012;57:2680–6.
12. Keswani RN. Single-balloon colonoscopy versus repeat standard colonoscopy for previous incomplete colonoscopy: a randomized, controlled trial. Gastrointest Endosc. 2011;73:507–12
13. Purchiaroni F, Conti S, Valerii G, et al. Use of enteroscope without the overtube in incomplete colonoscopies. Scand J Gastroenterol. 2020;55:100–4.

14. Schembre DB, Ross AS, Gluck MN, et al. Spiral overtube-assisted colonoscopy after incomplete colonoscopy in the redundant colon. Gastrointest Endosc. 2011;73:515–9.
15. Franco DL, Leighton JA, Gurudu SR. Approach to incomplete colonoscopy: new techniques and technologies. Gastroenterol Hepatol (N Y). 2017;13:476–83.

Other Small Bowel Endoscopies

6

Bong Min Ko, Hyun Jung Lee, and Jae Jun Park

Keywords
Push enteroscopy Proximal jejunum Intraoperative enteroscopy Small bowel bleedingPolyposis Spiral enteroscopy Motorized spiral enteroscopy Device-assisted enteroscopy

6.1 Push Enteroscopy

6.1.1 Introduction

Push enteroscopy is a method of examining the proximal jejunum using a specially designed enteroscope or a colonoscope with or without an overtube [1]. Its procedure is similar to that of the upper gastrointestinal endoscopy wherein the endoscopist manipulates the endoscope and inserts it while observing the gastrointestinal tract. Advantageously, push enteroscopy using a colonoscope can be readily performed without special training.

B. M. Ko (✉)
Division of Gastroenterology, Sunchunhyang University College of Medicine, Asan, South Korea
e-mail: kopa9445@schmc.ac.kr

H. J. Lee
Seoul National University College of Medicine, Seoul, South Korea
e-mail: guswjd80@snu.ac.kr

J. J. Park
Department of Gastroenterology, Yonsei University College of Medicine, Seoul, South Korea
e-mail: jaejpark@yuhs.ac

J.-J. Park et al. (eds.), *Balloon-Assisted Enteroscopy*,
https://doi.org/10.1007/978-981-95-2445-7_6

6.1.2 Indication

This procedure is performed for suspected lesions in the distal duodenum, proximal jejunum, or the terminal 10–15 cm of the ileum for diagnostic or therapeutic purposes (Figs. 6.1, 6.2, and 6.3).

6.1.3 Preparation and Procedure

1. Various endoscopes, including colonoscope and enteroscope, can be used for the procedure.
2. The preparation is similar to that of the upper gastrointestinal endoscopy.
3. CO_2 insufflation can reduce patient discomfort.
4. Using a commercially available sliding tube can prevent the endoscope from forming large loops in the stomach during insertion.

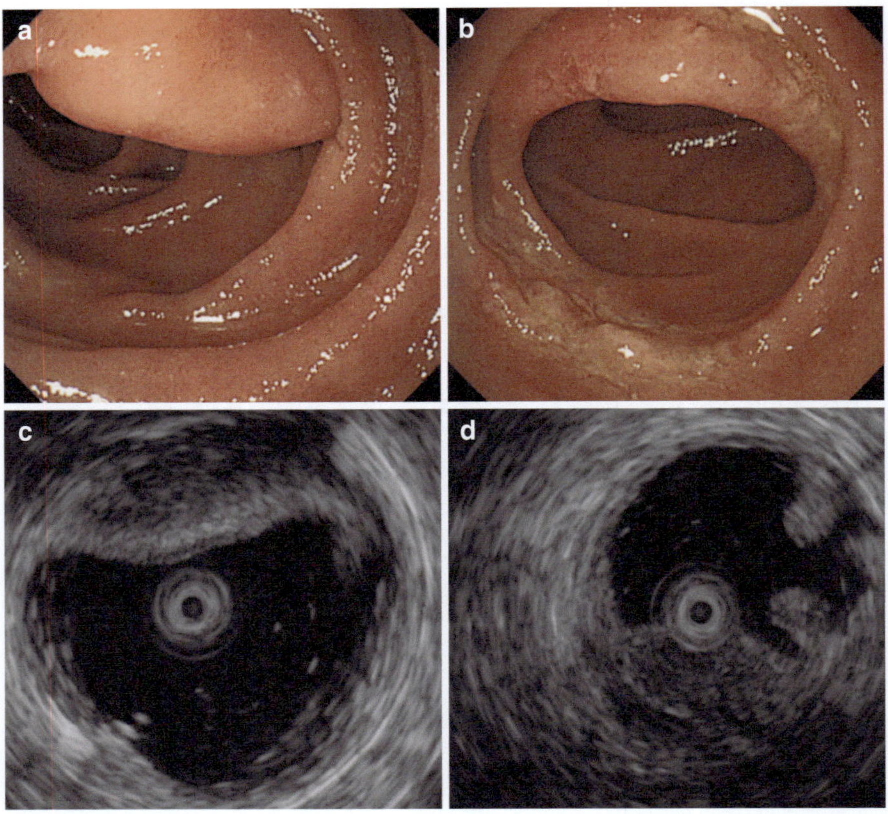

Fig. 6.1 Small intestinal amyloidosis. (**a**, **b**) Push enteroscopy findings. (**c**, **d**) Endoscopic ultrasonography findings using push enteroscopy

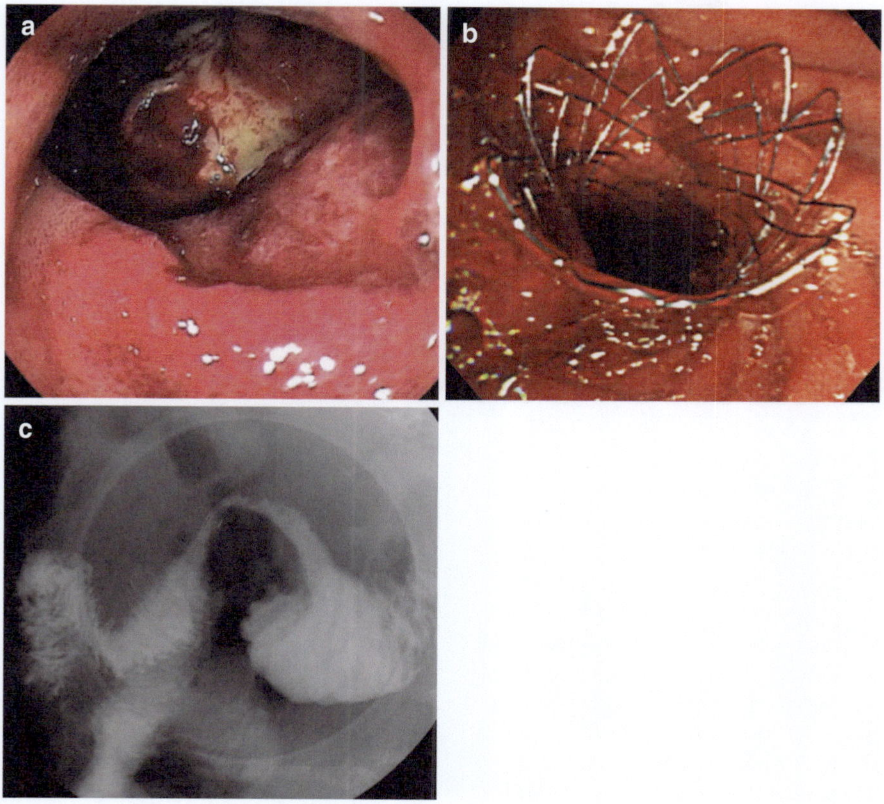

Fig. 6.2 Jejunal cancer-causing small intestinal obstruction. (**a**) Double-balloon enteroscopy finding. (**b**) Stent insertion using push enteroscopy. (**c**) Fluoroscopic findings

5. The endoscope is inserted into the small intestine as far as possible until restriction is noted.
6. Torque and withdrawal are repeated to reduce loop formation, thereby advancing the endoscope.
7. If the endoscope cannot advance further, the endoscopist may change patient's position and press the abdomen to facilitate insertion.
8. When using a variable stiffness colonoscope, the endoscopist reinforces the device to further advance it.
9. Fluoroscopy helps reduce the loops, identify the endoscope's position, and guide the direction of insertion.
10. Using an overtube can result in air leakage during insufflation and liquid discharge through the tube's opening.

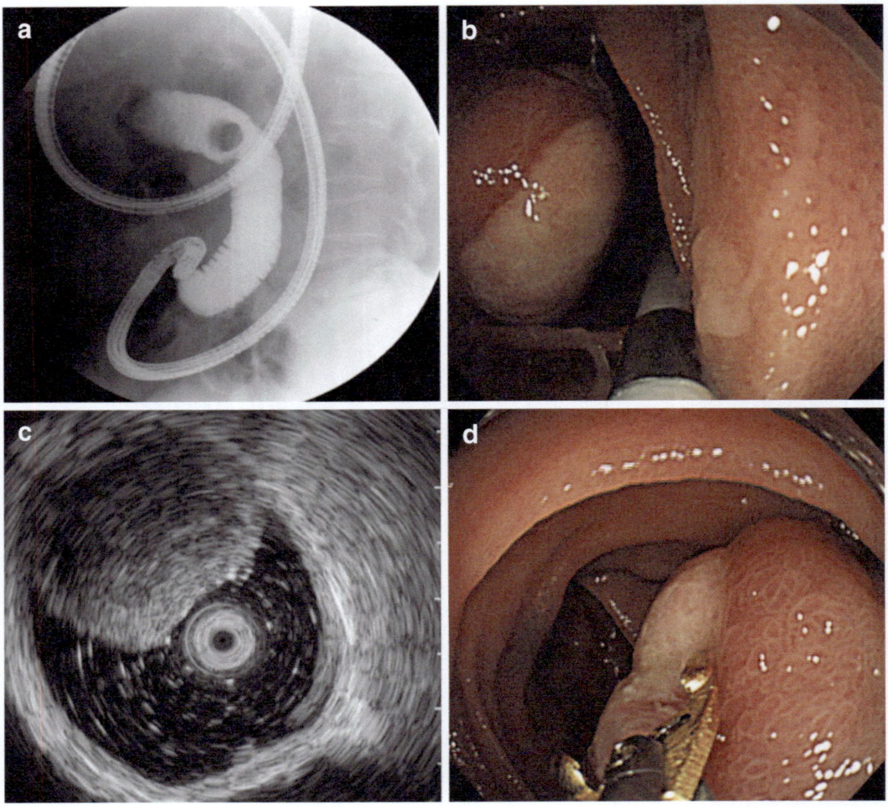

Fig. 6.3 Submucosal tumor of the small intestine. (**a**) Submucosal tumor of the small intestine detected via fluoroscopy. (**b**) Insertion using push enteroscopy with a catheter. (**c**) Ultrasonographic findings using push enteroscopy. (**d**) Biopsy using push enteroscopy

6.1.4 Clinical Results and Complications

Push enteroscopy does not require special equipment or training and can use existing equipment. The preparation is similar to that of the upper gastrointestinal endoscopy. A specially designed enteroscope or a colonoscope may be used; however, the length of the endoscope does not allow deeper insertion or improve the diagnostic rate [2–4]. Nevertheless, a colonoscope reportedly can reach 40–60 cm from the ligament of Treitz [5, 6]. Overtubes, which may cause discomfort, are not routinely used, but a commercially available small-bowel enteroscopy overtube can be employed if necessary. The diagnostic yield of push enteroscopy for obscure gastrointestinal bleeding is 20–80% [7]. Overall, push enteroscopy is considered safe [2]. Complications associated with push enteroscopy using a colonoscope often arise from the overtube and include mucosal stripping, parotid swelling, cardiopulmonary abnormalities, pancreatitis, and perforation; nonetheless, the reported complication rate is only 1% [8–10].

6.2 Intraoperative Enteroscopy

6.2.1 Introduction

Intraoperative enteroscopy is the most invasive form of enteroscopy, involving the use of an enteroscope to examine the small bowel during laparotomy. Historically, it was considered a standard diagnostic technique for a comprehensive evaluation of the small bowel, alongside push enteroscopy, ropeway enteroscopy, and sonde enteroscopy. However, its use has declined due to concerns about morbidity and mortality, along with the advancement of noninvasive imaging techniques and the introduction of capsule endoscopy and device-assisted enteroscopy. This study will explore the indications for intraoperative enteroscopy, the procedure itself, and its clinical outcomes.

6.2.2 Indication

6.2.2.1 Indications [11]

① Small Bowel Bleeding

Current guidelines recommend capsule endoscopy or device-assisted enteroscopy as the initial procedure for suspected small bowel bleeding after negative upper endoscopy and colonoscopy results [12]. Intraoperative enteroscopy should be considered for patients with recurrent bleeding who require multiple transfusions or hospitalizations after thorough negative evaluations using capsule endoscopy and device-assisted enteroscopy, or when lesions cannot be assessed or treated effectively with device-assisted enteroscopy.

② Crohn's Disease

Intraoperative enteroscopy is used to assess the extent and severity of inflammation and strictures in Crohn's disease patients that may require surgical intervention. This combined surgical and enteroscopic approach allows for the management of multiple small bowel strictures during the procedure [13].

③ Small Bowel Tumors and Polyposis

In Peutz–Jeghers syndrome, intraoperative enteroscopy helps clear polyps, preventing complications like intussusception or obstruction and reducing the need for repeated laparotomies. It can also be used to remove small bowel polyps in patients with familial adenomatous polyposis, particularly those who have had a Whipple procedure with a Roux-en-Y anastomosis. Furthermore, intraoperative enteroscopy aids in the diagnosis and localization of suspected small bowel tumors, including neuroendocrine tumors, adenocarcinomas, or lymphomas.

6.2.2.2 Contraindications

Intraoperative enteroscopy is typically performed under general anesthesia in the operating room, making it feasible when general endoscopic examination is possible. However, it is contraindicated in patients with severe cardiovascular or respiratory conditions or poor overall health or when the risks of the procedure outweigh the potential benefits. It is also contraindicated if the patient cannot provide adequate cooperation or consent or if a perforated viscus is suspected or known [14].

6.2.3 Technique

The procedure for intraoperative enteroscopy involves abdominal exploration followed by enteroscopy, which can be performed via a peroral, transanal, or surgically created enterotomy approach. Pediatric colonoscopes and enteroscopes are typically preferred, although gastroscopes and colonoscopes may also be used depending on the endoscopist's preference (Fig. 6.4) [15].

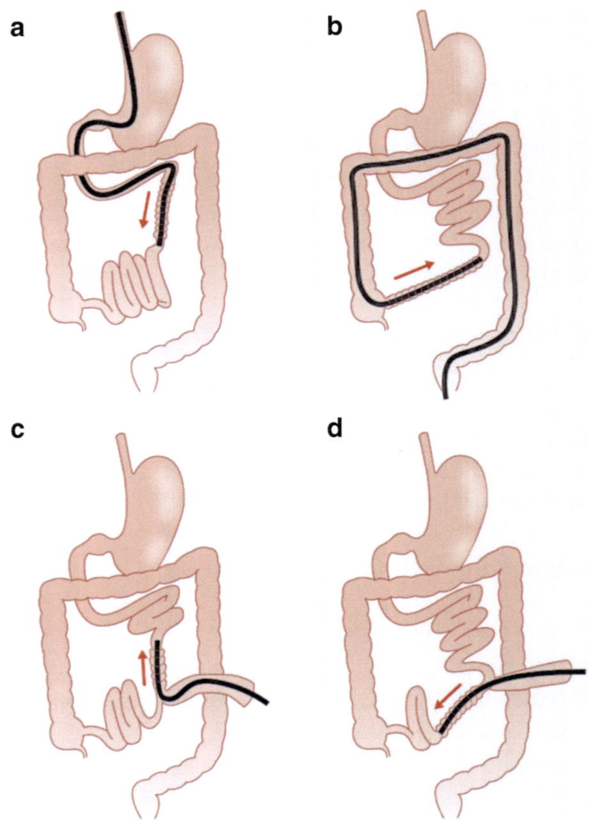

Fig. 6.4 Approaches to intraoperative enteroscopy. (**a**) Peroral. (**b**) Transanal. (**c**, **d**) Enterotomy technique

6.2.3.1 Abdominal Exploration

Abdominal exploration is the initial step in intraoperative enteroscopy, typically performed through a midline laparotomy, though a laparoscopic approach has also been used. In patients with previous abdominal surgery, thorough adhesiolysis is crucial to prevent iatrogenic injuries that might be mistaken for vascular lesions during enteroscopy. Following this, a comprehensive surgical exploration of the abdomen is necessary to identify any macroscopic abnormalities. This includes visual inspection and palpation of the stomach, duodenum, and the entire length of both the large and the small intestines, often using the transillumination technique.

6.2.3.2 Intraoperative Enteroscopy Approaches

Intraoperative enteroscopy can be performed through peroral, transanal, or enterotomy sites, or by combining these techniques (Fig. 6.4) [16]. The enterotomy approach is the standard method, enabling full inspection of the small bowel while minimizing mucosal damage. The enteroscope is inserted through a mid-small bowel enterotomy, either secured by a circular suture around the incision or via a sterile laparoscopic plastic sheath temporarily sutured to the edges of the enterotomy. The peroral or transanal approaches are less invasive but have limitations, such as being more time-consuming and limiting complete visualization of the small bowel. When using the transoral approach, an overtube may help prevent looping of the enteroscope in the stomach and duodenum. An additional enterotomy may also be necessary to avoid overdistension when reaching the terminal ileum.

6.2.3.3 Practical Aspects

Intraoperative enteroscopy requires a dual examination: the endoscopist uses the enteroscope internally, while the surgeon performs an external examination with transillumination. The "air-trapping" technique, where a segment of the bowel is pinched to trap air and to keep the lumen open, helps achieve optimal mucosal visualization. Unlike colonoscopy, observing the mucosa during advancement of the enteroscope—rather than during withdrawal—prevents misinterpretation of mucosal damage as vascular lesions. Any identified lesions are marked with sutures on the serosal surface for potential future resection if enteroscopic treatment is not possible. CO_2 insufflation is preferred over air insufflation to reduce bowel distension, and proper desufflation is essential after the procedure.

6.2.4 Clinical Outcomes

6.2.4.1 Diagnostic and Therapeutic Yield

Complete enteroscopy success rates range from 57% to 100%. A review of 16 studies found a diagnostic yield of 79% and a therapeutic yield of 74% [16]. Vascular lesions (61%) were the most commonly identified bleeding sources, followed by ulcers (19%), tumors (10%), and diverticula (4%). Vascular lesions like angiodysplasia can be treated enteroscopically with argon plasma coagulation, while tumors, ulcers, or diverticula are marked with sutures and treated surgically. Rebleeding rates vary from 13% to 52%. In particular, intraoperative enteroscopy is valuable for patients with familial adenomatous polyposis, those who have undergone Roux-en-Y surgery, and those with Peutz–Jeghers syndrome, where previous surgeries and adhesions complicate full examination. It aids in polyp removal and lowers the risk of short bowel syndrome due to repeated bowel resections.

6.2.4.2 Complications

Complication rates vary from 1% to 50%, with mortality associated with the procedure or postoperative complications reaching as high as 18%. Surgical morbidities, occurring in up to 12.5% of cases, include mucosal lacerations, intramural hematomas, mesenteric hemorrhages, perforations, prolonged postoperative ileus, and wound infections. Medical complications have been reported in 4.6% of cases, including pneumonia, cardiovascular issues, pulmonary embolism, and azotemia [17].

6.2.5 Conclusion

With the advancements in capsule endoscopy and device-assisted enteroscopy, the use of intraoperative enteroscopy has significantly decreased, making careful patient selection based on preprocedural indications essential. Intraoperative enteroscopy is still indicated when small bowel lesions, identified in preoperative evaluations, are inaccessible or difficult to treat with device-assisted enteroscopy or cannot be localized during surgery. Given the procedure's invasive nature and associated risks, a multidisciplinary approach involving gastroenterology, surgery, and radiology is crucial for appropriate decision-making and management.

6.3 Spiral Enteroscopy

6.3.1 Introduction

The recent clinical guidelines established by multiple medical societies have emphasized the roles of small-bowel capsule endoscopy and enteroscopy in the diagnosis and the treatment of small-bowel diseases. Small-bowel enteroscopy provides direct access to small-bowel lesions, thereby allowing both tissue biopsy and therapeutic interventions. However, small-bowel enteroscopy is a technically challenging procedure, and several devices and techniques have been developed to facilitate endoscopic access to the deep small bowel. Among these, the double-balloon (Fujifilm, Tokyo, Japan) and single-balloon (Olympus Medical Systems Corporation, Tokyo, Japan) enteroscopy systems are the most commonly used small-bowel endoscopy devices. However, mastering the techniques involved remains challenging.

Meanwhile, the spiral enteroscopy system, which uses the Endo-Ease overtube (Spirus Medical, LLC, West Bridgewater, Massachusetts, the USA), is the most recently developed enteroscopic technology. The principle behind spiral enteroscopy is the conversion of the rotational energy of the spiral into a linear force, which draws the bowel over the endoscope. Recently, the motorized spiral enteroscopy system (Power Spiral Enteroscopy) has been developed. This system is a novel advancement that incorporates a motorized feature that allows endoscopists to control the rotation of the spiral overtube via an attached motor, which facilitates insertion. The diagnostic and therapeutic efficacy of these spiral enteroscopy systems are similar to those of the conventional balloon-assisted enteroscopy. Further, these systems have advantages. In particular, they are associated with an easier and more straightforward endoscopic manipulation.

6.3.2 Indications and Contraindications

6.3.2.1 Indications

The indications of small-intestine spiral enteroscopy are similar to those of balloon-assisted enteroscopy. Small-intestine spiral enteroscopy is indicated for patients requiring endoscopic examination of the small intestine, such as those with obscure gastrointestinal bleeding or suspected inflammatory bowel disease, and for those requiring therapeutic interventions such as polypectomy, hemostasis, and stricture dilation. Notably, compared with balloon-assisted enteroscopy, spiral enteroscopy is advantageous in maintaining endoscopic stability during histologic biopsy of the small intestine and endoscopic therapeutic procedures, such as argon plasma coagulation, clipping, polypectomy, and stricture dilation.

6.3.2.2 Contraindications

Spiral enteroscopy is contraindicated to patients who cannot tolerate general anesthesia or those with prolonged deep sedation. The other contraindications include suspected gastrointestinal perforation, uncontrolled coagulopathy, recent placement of a feeding jejunostomy tube, and pediatric age. Further contraindications to the transoral approach include esophageal or gastric varices, upper gastrointestinal strictures, deep mucosal lacerations, suspected eosinophilic esophagitis, and conditions causing difficulties in placing a mouthpiece.

The relative contraindications include conditions such as cervical disc herniation and inability to extend the neck. The contraindications to the transanal access include severe active inflammation of the colon and anorectal or colonic strictures. In addition, cautious consideration is required for patients with conditions that may involve intestinal strictures, those with a history of abdominal or pelvic surgery, those with an altered bowel anatomy, or pregnant women.

6.3.3 Preparation and Procedure

For pre-procedural bowel preparation, fasting from the night before is generally sufficient for the transoral approach. However, for the transanal approach, bowel cleansing similar to that required in colonoscopy is necessary. In case of manual spiral enteroscopy performed using the transoral approach, the procedure may be conducted either under general anesthesia or sedation, based on the institution's experience. In contrast, motorized spiral enterostomy is typically performed under general anesthesia. For the transanal approach, both manual and motorized spiral enteroscopy procedures are generally performed with sedation.

6.3.4 Manual Spiral Enteroscopy

In 2005, Akerman and Cantero introduced manual spiral enteroscopy to facilitate deep small-bowel visualization [18]. This device utilizes an entirely new concept, advancing by engaging the bowel with an actively rotating instrumentation shaft, not by pushing force. The principle behind this method is to draw the intestine over the endoscope by converting rotational energy into linear force, thereby enabling deeper endoscope insertion. In the initial report of Akerman and Cantero, an overtube with spiral projections (Endo-Ease Discovery SB overtube) and a pediatric colonoscope were used [18]. The length of the overtube is 118 cm, and the overtube has a 5-mm high spiral over the distal 21-cm segment. This overtube could be mounted on endoscopes with diameters up to 9.4 mm. Later iterations of the overtube were refined with a smaller diameter and softer spirals.

During the procedure, a lubricant is applied to the inside of the spiral overtube, which is then locked in place 22 cm from the endoscope's distal tip. This section of the endoscope without the overtube allows a smoother passage via the upper gastrointestinal tract to the ligament of Treitz. Once it passed the ligament of Treitz, the spiral overtube is applied via clockwise rotation to engage the small bowel and fold it onto the endoscope, thereby facilitating a deeper insertion into the small intestine. When further rotation of the overtube can no longer advance the bowel onto the endoscope, the overtube is unlocked from the endoscope, thereby allowing it to advance maximally into the small intestine. Retrieval of the endoscope is achieved by slowly rotating the overtube counterclockwise [18].

6.3.5 Motorized Spiral Enteroscopy

A novel motorized spiral enteroscope (Olympus Medical Systems Corporation, Tokyo, Japan) was introduced in 2015 [19]. The length and diameter of the motorized spiral enteroscope are 168 cm (Fig. 6.5a, b) and 12.8 mm, respectively. Moreover, it has a 3.2-mm working channel, which is compatible with standard colonoscopic accessories. This enteroscope incorporates a built-in motor that drives the rotation of the spiral overtube, which is controlled by a foot pedal (Fig. 6.5c). The pedal has two parts: the forward pedal, which rotates the spiral overtube clockwise, folding the intestine onto the overtube to enable endoscopic advancement, and the reverse pedal, which releases the folded intestine, thereby allowing it to disengage from the endoscope.

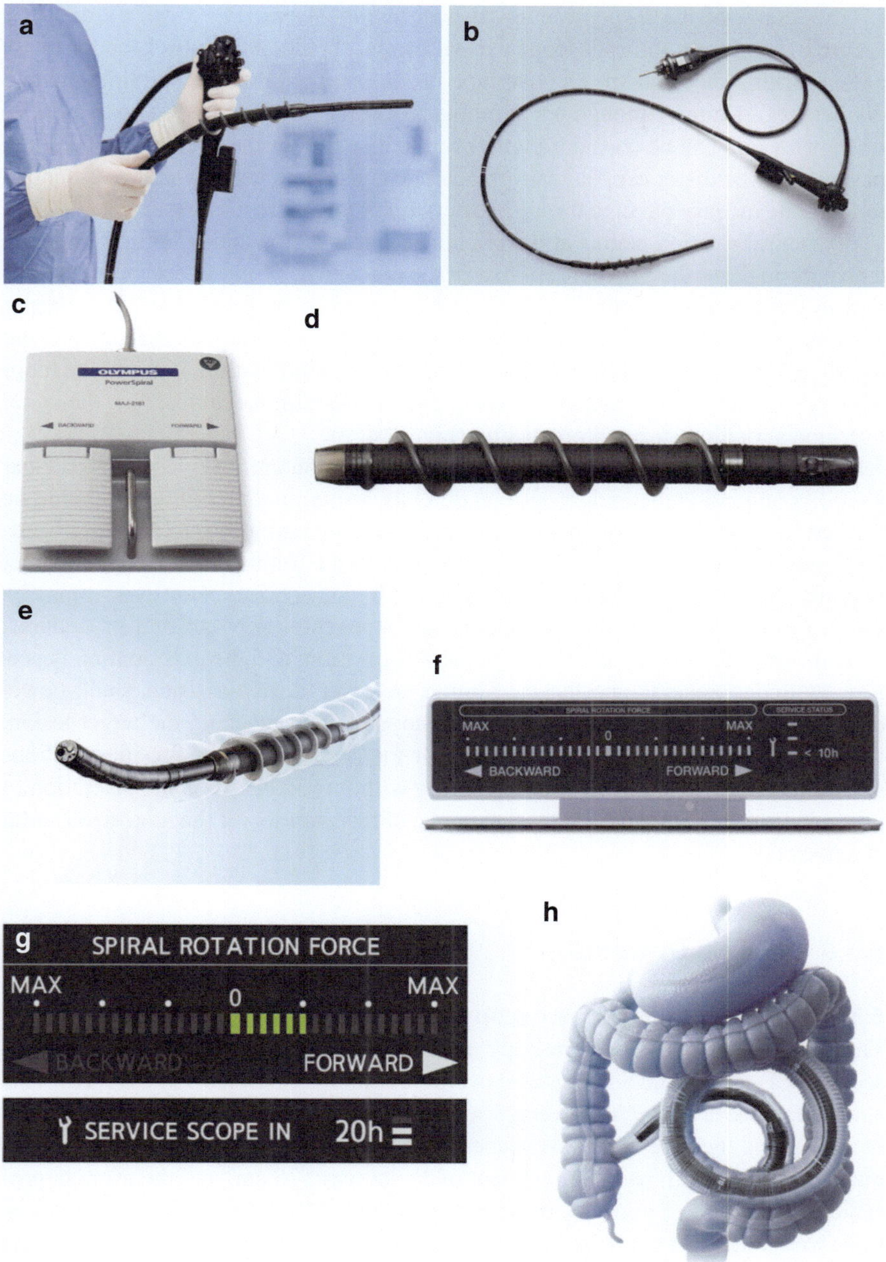

Fig. 6.5 Motorized spiral enteroscopy. (**a**, **b**) Motorized spiral enteroscopy. (**c**) Foot pedal for the rotational control of the spiral overtube. (**d**) Overtube for motorized spiral enteroscopy. (**e**) Image of the motorized spiral enteroscopy overtube mounted on the endoscope. (**f**) Endoscope load pressure gauge. (**g**) Endoscope load pressure gauge during forward insertion. (**h**) Schematic of the transoral insertion approach for motorized spiral enteroscopy

The length of the disposable spiral overtube is 24 cm (Fig. 6.5d, e), and it is secured 16 cm from the endoscope's distal tip (just behind the control section) with a dual locking mechanism. The overtube is equipped with rubber spiral fins with a diameter of 31 mm. Although not a routine procedure, graded dilation up to approximately 18 mm can be considered prior to the insertion of the overtube to facilitate passage via the upper esophageal sphincter. The patient's neck should be extended to facilitate an easy passage through the cricopharyngeal region.

The spiral rotation begins at the cricopharyngeal region and continues intermittently throughout the procedure. Forward advancement of the endoscope, in addition to the rotational control of the spiral overtube, is performed to reach deeper sections of the small intestine. A force gauge is also a safety feature that can prevent intestinal damage caused by excessive force during manipulation. If excessive looping or distal bowel obstruction creates undue pressure on the endoscope, the spiral overtube's rotation stops automatically (Fig. 6.5f, g).

During insertion, carbon dioxide and water infusion are used to maintain clear visibility and guide the endoscope's path. Only a small volume of water should be infused to facilitate endoscopic advancement when passing through sharply bending sections. Excessive water infusion may inhibit the folding of the intestinal tract over the spiral overtube. Fluoroscopy is generally unnecessary. However, it may be used in rare cases to validate the endoscope's position. For transoral procedures, patients are placed in the left lateral decubitus position, and the examination is performed under general anesthesia. Similar to other device-assisted small-bowel enteroscopy methods, insertion is usually stopped upon reaching the target lesion, which is the point of maximal insertion, or the cecum. Therapeutic interventions and biopsies are generally performed during withdrawal, based on the discretion of the endoscopist. Figure 6.5h shows an image of the insertion of the motorized spiral enteroscope.

6.3.6 Clinical Outcomes

6.3.6.1 Manual Spiral Enteroscopy

The first report on spiral enteroscopy used a system combining a pediatric colonoscope (PCF-140 L) and a specialized overtube (Endo-Ease Discovery SB) [18]. This study included 27 patients (average age: 44 years) with obscure gastrointestinal bleeding, and the procedure was successfully completed in 93% of cases [18]. The mean insertion depth past the ligament of Treitz was 176 cm, and the average procedure time was 36.5 min. The diagnostic yield was 33%, and significant complications were not observed. Although this early spiral enteroscope was larger than the later commercial models, its stability and efficacy are similar to those of the spiral enteroscopy technique [18].

Subsequently, the Discovery SB overtube was modified to accommodate slimmer 200-cm double- and single-balloon enteroscopes from Fujinon and Olympus. In a prospective study involving 75 patients [20], a comparison was made between the 200-cm, 9.4-mm Fujinon EN-450 T5 and the 9.2-mm Olympus SIF-Q180. The

Fujinon group included 50 patients with an average age of 46.2 years. Meanwhile, the Olympus group comprised 25 patients, with an average age 45 years. The most common indication was obscure gastrointestinal bleeding (n = 58), followed by diarrhea (n = 12) and abdominal pain (n = 5). The average estimated insertion depths past the ligament of Treitz were 243 cm in the Fujinon group and 256 cm in the Olympus group. In the Fujinon group, the average time to reach the maximum depth was 18.7 min, with a total procedure time of 26.1 min and a diagnostic yield of 22%. The Olympus group had similar outcomes, with total procedure times of 16.2 and 26.1 min and a diagnostic yield of 32%. Neither of the groups did not present with significant complications, and there were no statistically significant differences between them. Compared with the prototype, the newly designed Discovery SB overtube had a better insertion depth and lower procedure time.

In another prospective multicenter study involving 149 patients with an average age of 68 years, the Discovery SB overtube was successfully used in 93% of cases [21]. The mean insertion depth past the ligament of Treitz was 250.3 cm, with a time to reach maximum depth of 35.4 min and a total procedure time of 45 min. The diagnostic yield was 65.2%, and severe complications were not recorded. All endoscopists participating in the study had prior experience with balloon-assisted enteroscopy. Moreover, they reported that spiral enteroscopy had superior safety during interventional procedures. The overall clinical outcomes were similar to those reported in other deep small-bowel enteroscopy studies.

Khashab et al. conducted a retrospective study comparing single-balloon enteroscopy and spiral enteroscopy, with a total of 105 procedures performed on 92 patients at a single institution [22]. This study included 52 patients in the single-balloon enteroscopy group and 53 in the spiral enteroscopy group, with an average age of 55 years. The mean total procedure times of single-balloon enteroscopy and spiral enteroscopy were 53 and 47 min, respectively. The maximum insertion depths past the ligament of Treitz were 222 cm in single-balloon enteroscopy and 301 cm in spiral enteroscopy, with diagnostic yields of 58% and 43.3%, respectively. One patient in the single-balloon enteroscopy group developed small-bowel perforation. In this first comparative study, spiral enteroscopy had a statistically significant advantage in terms of maximum small-bowel insertion depth over single-balloon enteroscopy, without significant difference in diagnostic yield or procedure time between the two groups. Schembre et al. compared double-balloon enteroscopy and spiral enteroscopy in 57 patients (average age: 65 years) with obscure gastrointestinal bleeding [23]. Capsule endoscopy was performed before double-balloon enteroscopy in 53% of cases and before spiral enteroscopy in 70% of cases. The spiral enteroscopy group had a shorter total procedure time than the double-balloon enteroscopy group (59 vs. 77 min). Meanwhile, the two groups had similar diagnostic yields (65% vs. 70%). None of the patients in the two groups developed severe complications. Based on this study, both procedures are effective in diagnosing and treating obscure gastrointestinal bleeding, with spiral enteroscopy being advantageous due to its shorter procedure times.

Subsequently, prospective studies have compared spiral enteroscopy and balloon-assisted enteroscopy. For example, May et al. conducted a prospective crossover study comparing double-balloon enteroscopy and spiral enteroscopy in 18 patients (average age: 69 years) [24]. This study found that double-balloon enteroscopy and spiral enteroscopy differed in terms of total procedure time and maximum insertion depth. In particular, spiral enteroscopy had a shorter total procedure time than double-balloon enteroscopy (43 vs. 65 min). Meanwhile, double-balloon enteroscopy had a greater maximum insertion depth than spiral enteroscopy (250 vs. 310 cm). Although the small sample size limited definitive conclusions, the study showed that each enteroscopy technique has unique advantages [24].

Despott et al. conducted another prospective study on 15 patients. This research first performed spiral enteroscopy to the maximum insertion depth, marking this point before conducting double-balloon enteroscopy [25]. In 93% (14 of 15) of cases, double-balloon enteroscopy surpassed the maximum insertion depth achieved by spiral enteroscopy, with median insertion depths of 175 and 265 cm in spiral and double-balloon enteroscopy, respectively ($p = 0.004$). However, spiral enteroscopy had a shorter median time to reach the maximum depth than double-balloon enteroscopy (24 vs. 45 min, $p = 0.0005$). Moreover, the median time to reach the marked location in 14 patients did not significantly differ between the two techniques ($p = 0.28$). Although this study has a small sample size, it revealed that double-balloon enteroscopy has a significantly deeper insertion depth than the spiral enteroscopy. Double-balloon enteroscopy had a longer overall procedure time than spiral enteroscopy. However, the time to reach the same insertion depth was similar between the two methods.

In summary, compared with the traditional balloon-assisted enteroscopy, manual spiral enteroscopy is advantageous as it has a shorter procedure time and more stable endoscopic positioning during therapeutic interventions. Due to limited data, it is challenging to achieve definitive conclusions about the maximum insertion depth of double-balloon enteroscopy unlike that of single-balloon enteroscopy. However, previous studies have revealed that spiral enteroscopy has a shorter insertion depth than the double-balloon enteroscopy.

6.3.6.2 Transanal Spiral Enteroscopy

Previous reports on the transanal access in spiral enteroscopy are limited. The procedure involves advancing the endoscope and Discovery SB overtube through the transanal route to reach the terminal ileum. Once there, clockwise rotation of the overtube folds the small intestine onto the overtube, thereby allowing a deeper insertion. In the transanal approach, similar to the transoral approach, the endoscope is withdrawn by rotating the overtube counterclockwise.

A retrospective study analyzed the feasibility of the transanal approach for evaluating small-bowel diseases using spiral enteroscopy in six patients with a mean age of 50 years [26]. In this research, the indications included obscure gastrointestinal bleeding ($n = 2$), polyps ($n = 1$), cystic fibrosis with associated strictures ($n = 1$), small-bowel obstruction ($n = 1$), and abnormal findings on abdominal CT scan ($n = 1$). The mean maximum insertion depth from the ileocecal valve was 75 cm, with an average total procedure time of 52 min and a diagnostic yield of 67%. No complications were reported. This study revealed that the transanal approach for spiral enteroscopy was technically feasible and had a shorter procedure time than other enteroscopy methods, based on the researchers' prior experience with small-bowel endoscopy. In another study on 22 patients (mean age: 64 years), the clinical outcomes of transanal spiral enteroscopy were evaluated [27]. The indications were obscure gastrointestinal bleeding (77.3%), Crohn's disease (18.2%), and tumors (4.5%). The mean maximum insertion depth from the ileocecal valve was 100 cm, with an average procedure time of 49.6 min and a diagnostic yield of 45.4%. No significant procedure-related complications were noted. Based on this study, the feasibility of transanal spiral enteroscopy was comparable to that of double-balloon enteroscopy, with the added benefit of shorter procedure times. Further, the spiral overtube contributed to stable endoscopic manipulation, thereby effectively facilitating therapeutic interventions.

6.3.6.3 Endoscopic Retrograde Cholangiopancreatography Assisted by Spiral Enteroscopy in Patients with an Altered Anatomical Bowel Structure After Surgery

Endoscopic retrograde cholangiopancreatography (ERCP) is challenging to perform in patients with surgically altered anatomical bowel structures, as reaching the papilla is difficult with conventional endoscopy. In such cases, spiral enteroscopy can be an alternative approach to access the papilla, thereby facilitating diagnostic and therapeutic ERCP.

A previous study has evaluated the clinical outcomes of spiral enteroscopy-assisted ERCP in patients with an altered anatomy caused by Roux-en-Y gastric bypass ($n = 7$) and standard Roux-en-Y surgery ($n = 2$) [28]. The diagnostic success rate was 89%, with an average total procedure time of 65 min and an average time to reach the pancreatobiliary anastomosis of 27 min. Another study compared spiral enteroscopy-assisted ERCP and single-balloon enteroscopy-assisted ERCP in 54 ERCP cases in 34 patients who underwent Roux-en-Y surgery [29]. Spiral enteroscopy has some advantages over single-balloon enteroscopy in terms of procedure time and stability. However, both methods are similar in terms of diagnostic and therapeutic efficacy [29].

Although limited, current studies have revealed that spiral enteroscopy-assisted ERCP can be an alternative diagnostic and treatment strategy in patients with an altered bowel anatomy after surgery. Compared with balloon-assisted enteroscopy, spiral enteroscopy is safe and feasible in patients with modified anatomical structures, similar to other gastrointestinal conditions based on previous clinical reports. In addition, it may be advantageous due to its shorter procedure time and relatively superior stability in endoscopic manipulation. Nevertheless, further prospective studies should be performed to expand these findings.

6.3.6.4 Motorized Spiral Enteroscopy

The first prospective feasibility study on motorized spiral enteroscopy was conducted on patients with suspected small-bowel disease who were candidates for transoral small-bowel enteroscopy [30]. This study primarily aimed to evaluate the diagnostic yield of transoral motorized spiral enteroscopy. Further, it secondarily aimed to assess technical success (defined as insertion at least up to the ligament of Treitz) rate, maximum insertion depth, median insertion time, therapeutic interventions, and adverse events. Over 30 months, 132 patients (74 men, 58 women; mean age: 68 [range: 20–100] years) at two tertiary medical centers underwent 140 procedures under general anesthesia. The overall diagnostic yield was 74.2%, and therapeutic endoscopic procedures were performed in 68.2% of cases. In addition, the technical success rate was 97%, with a median maximum insertion depth of 450 (range: 0–600) cm and a median insertion time of 25 (range: 3–122) min. Complete visualization of the small intestine up to the cecum using the transoral access was achieved in 14 (10.6%) cases. Based on these results, the transoral approach motorized spiral enteroscopy is useful for patients with small-intestine disorders.

Another study evaluated the total enteroscopy rate in patients with indications for complete small-bowel examination. In this research, transoral motorized spiral enteroscopy was initially performed. Then, transanal motorized spiral enteroscopy was conducted if total small-bowel visualization was not achieved using the transoral route alone [31]. The primary outcome was the total enteroscopy rate. This study included 30 patients (14 men, 16 women; median age: 64 [range: 37–100] years). The technical success rate of transoral motorized spiral enteroscopy (defined as insertion beyond the ligament of Treitz) and transanal motorized spiral enteroscopy (defined as insertion beyond the ileocecal valve) was 100%. The total enteroscopy rate was 70%, which was achieved using the transoral access alone in 16.6% of cases and by combining the transoral and transanal access in 53.4% of cases. The median maximum insertion depth from the ligament of Treitz during the transoral access was 490 (range: 160–600) cm, with a median insertion time of 26 (range: 15–110) min. For the transanal approach, the median maximum insertion depth beyond the ileocecal valve was 120 (range: 40–600) cm, with a median insertion time of 17 (range: 1–68) min. The overall diagnostic yield and therapeutic intervention rates were 80% and 86.7%, respectively. In this study, motorized spiral enteroscopy achieved a complete small-intestine examination rate of 70%, which is significantly higher than that of other device-assisted enteroscopy procedures. Therefore, combining oral and transanal approaches facilitated the observation of the whole small intestine in a substantial number of patients. Further, the median time to maximum insertion was within 30 min for both the transoral and the transanal routes, thereby underscoring the advantage of rapid examination with motorized spiral enteroscopy.

A recent randomized controlled trial compared motorized spiral enteroscopy and single-balloon enteroscopy in patients with small-bowel disorders [32]. Results showed that motorized spiral enteroscopy had a significantly higher total enteroscopy rate than SBE (71.4% vs 10.8%) ($p < 0.0001$). Further, motorized spiral enteroscopy had a shorter total procedure time (58.17 ± 21.5 vs. 114.2 ± 33.5 min, $p < 0.0001$) and a higher diagnostic yield (80% vs. 62.1%, $p = 0.096$) than single-balloon enteroscopy. Obscure gastrointestinal bleeding (48%) was the most common indication for the procedures. Based on these findings, compared with SBE, motorized spiral enteroscopy is a more efficient and effective method for small-bowel examination.

6.3.7 Complications of Spiral Enteroscopy

6.3.7.1 Manual Spiral Enteroscopy

The incidence of major complications associated with spiral enteroscopy is relatively low and comparable to that of balloon-assisted enteroscopy. A large retrospective study analyzed complications in 2950 patients who underwent spiral enteroscopy. Results showed that the incidence rate of severe complications was 0.3%. The most common severe complication was small-bowel perforation, which occurred in 0.27% (8 of 2950) patients, all of whom required surgical treatment [32]. There were no deaths caused by major complications, and none of the patients ($n = 2950$) developed acute pancreatitis.

In another study examining the complications of spiral enteroscopy in 61 elderly patients with comorbidities (mean age: 65.4 years), the average procedure time was 41 min, and visualization beyond the ligament of Treitz was achieved in 92% of cases, with a maximum insertion depth of 217.4 cm beyond the ligament [33]. Approximately 7% of cases involved mild complications. Meanwhile, major complications were not reported. Based on these findings, spiral enteroscopy can be safely performed on elderly patients. In particular, spiral enteroscopy is associated with a potential risk of adverse effects such as esophageal mucosal injury caused by the spiral-shaped overtube. Thus, caution should be observed during oral approach procedures.

6.3.7.2 Motorized Spiral Enteroscopy

In recent prospective studies, the overall complication rate of motorized spiral enteroscopy was 14.4%. There were two (1.5%) cases of major complications, specifically delayed perforation and Mallory-Weiss syndrome [30]. In another report, 4 of 14 patients who underwent powered spiral enteroscopy developed serious complications ($n = 3$, hypothermia and $n = 1$, pancreatitis). All patients recovered without any sequelae [34, 35]. In a study evaluating the total enteroscopy rate using both the transoral and the transanal access with motorized spiral enteroscopy, the overall complication rate was 16.7%. No major complications were observed. Similarly, a recent randomized controlled trial has shown that motorized spiral enteroscopy and single-balloon enteroscopy had similar safety profiles in patients with small-bowel disorders [32]. Approximately 8.5% of the patients who underwent motorized spiral enteroscopy and 5.4% of patients who underwent single-balloon enteroscopy developed minor adverse events.

However, motorized spiral enteroscopy was withdrawn from the global market in July 2023 after an urgent safety notification about esophageal injuries. These adverse events primarily occurred during the withdrawal phase. They were caused by the automated progression of the large spiral segment, which led to esophageal lacerations and, in rare cases, perforations. This underscores the importance of refining this technology to enhance safety while preserving its clinical benefits.

6.3.8 Conclusion

Various studies have shown that spiral enteroscopy is a valuable tool for evaluating the deep small intestine. This technique is a safe and effective endoscopic method, with a complication rate comparable to that of balloon-assisted enteroscopy. The diagnostic and therapeutic efficacy of spiral enteroscopy was similar to that of other device-assisted enteroscopy methods. In addition, spiral enteroscopy has a shorter procedure time and a better stability during endoscope manipulation compared with the conventional balloon-assisted enteroscopy. Therefore, it is advantageous when used in different therapeutic procedures.

Further, with the recent introduction of motorized spiral enteroscopy, the procedure has achieved significantly high rates of complete small-bowel visualization. However, the recent withdrawal of motorized spiral enteroscopy from the global market due to safety concerns, including esophageal injuries and rare perforations, underscores the urgent need for technological refinements to address these issues. Spiral enteroscopy has several advantages over balloon-assisted techniques. However, its reintroduction and potential expansion, which are important in device-assisted small-bowel endoscopy, will depend on the resolution of safety concerns and achievement of regulatory approval.

References

1. Committee AT, Chauhan SS, Manfredi MA, et al. Enteroscopy. Gastrointest Endosc. 2015;82:975–90.
2. Eisen GM, Dominitz JA, Faigel DO, et al. Enteroscopy. Gastrointest Endosc. 2001;53:871–3.
3. Benz C, Jakobs R, Riemann JF. Do we need the overtube for push-enteroscopy? Endoscopy. 2001;33:658–61.
4. Taylor AC, Chen RY, Desmond PV. Use of an overtube for enteroscopy—does it increase depth of insertion? A prospective study of enteroscopy with and without an overtube. Endoscopy. 2001;33:227–30.
5. Benz C, Jakobs R, Riemann JF. Does the insertion depth in push enteroscopy depend on the working length of the enteroscope? Endoscopy. 2002;34:543–5.
6. Sharma BC, Bhasin DK, Makharia G, et al. Diagnostic value of push-type enteroscopy: a report from India. Am J Gastroenterol. 2000;95:137–40.
7. Raju GS, Gerson L, Das A, et al. American Gastroenterological Association (AGA) institute technical review on obscure gastrointestinal bleeding. Gastroenterology. 2007;133:1697–717.
8. Oates BC, Morris AI. Enteroscopy. Curr Opin Gastroenterol. 2000;16:121–5.
9. Akerman PA, Cantero D. Spiral enteroscopy and push enteroscopy. Gastrointest Endosc Clin N Am. 2009;19:357–69.
10. Asge Technology C, DiSario JA, Petersen BT, et al. Enteroscopes. Gastrointest Endosc. 2007;66:872–80.
11. Schulz HJ, Schmidt H. Intraoperative enteroscopy. Gastrointest Endosc Clin N Am. 2009;19:371–9.
12. Gerson LB, Fidler JL, Cave DR, et al. ACG clinical guideline: diagnosis and management of small bowel bleeding. Am J Gastroenterol. 2015;110:1265–87.
13. Guo Q. Intraoperative endoscopic interventions of inflammatory bowel disease. Gastrointest Endosc Clin N Am. 2022;32:817–27.

14. Early DS, Ben-Menachem T, Decker GA, et al. Appropriate use of GI endoscopy. Gastrointest Endosc. 2012;75:1127–31.
15. Bonnet S, Douard R, Malamut G, et al. Intraoperative enteroscopy in the management of obscure gastrointestinal bleeding. Dig Liver Dis. 2013;45:277–84.
16. Voron T, Rahmi G, Bonnet S, et al. Intraoperative enteroscopy: is there still a role? Gastrointest Endosc Clin N Am. 2017;27:153–70.
17. Chauhan SS, Manfredi MA, Abu Dayyeh BK, et al. Enteroscopy. Gastrointest Endosc. 2015;82:975–90.
18. Akerman PA, Agrawal D, Chen W, Cantero D, Avila J, Pangtay J. Spiral enteroscopy: a novel method of enteroscopy by using the endo-ease discovery SB overtube and a pediatric colonoscope. Gastrointest Endosc. 2009;69:327–32.
19. Neuhaus H, Beyna T, Schneider M, Devière J. Novel motorized spiral enteroscopy: first clinical case. VideoGIE. 2016;1:32–3.
20. Akerman PA, Cantero D. Single physician technique for spiral enteroscopy. Gastrointest Endosc Clin N Am. 2009;19(3):357–69.
21. Morgan D, Upchurch B, Draganov P, et al. Spiral enteroscopy: prospective U.S. multicenter study in patients with small-bowel disorders. Gastrointest Endosc. 2010;72:992–8.
22. Khashab MA, Lennon AM, Dunbar KB, et al. A comparative evaluation of single-balloon enteroscopy and spiral enteroscopy for patients with mid-gut disorders. Gastrointest Endosc. 2010;72:766–72.
23. Schembre DS, Ross AM. Yield of antegrade double balloon versus spiral enteroscopy for obscure bleeding. Gastrointest Endosc. 2009;69:AB193.
24. May A, Manner H, Aschmoneit I, Ell C. Prospective, cross-over, single-center trial comparing oral double-balloon enteroscopy and oral spiral enteroscopy in patients with suspected small-bowel vascular malformations. Endoscopy. 2011;43:477–83.
25. Despott EJ, Murino A, Bourikas L, Nakamura M, Ramachandra V, Fraser C. A prospective comparison of performance during back-to-back, anterograde manual spiral enteroscopy and double-balloon enteroscopy. Dig Liver Dis. 2015;47:395–400.
26. Lara LF, Singh S, Sreenarasimhaiah J. Initial experience with retrograde overtube-assisted enteroscopy using a spiral tip overtube. Proc (Bayl Univ Med Cent). 2010;23:130–3.
27. Nagula S, Gaidos J, Draganov PV, et al. Retrograde spiral enteroscopy: feasibility, success, and safety in a series of 22 patients. Gastrointest Endosc. 2011;74:699–702.
28. Akerman PA, Cantero D. Spiral enteroscopy ERCP in surgically altered gastrointestinal anatomy. Endoscopy. 2009;41:872–7.
29. Lennon AM, Kapoor S, Khashab M, et al. Spiral assisted ERCP is equivalent to single balloon assisted ERCP in patients with roux-en-Y anatomy. Dig Dis Sci. 2012;57:1391–8.
30. Beyna T, Arvanitakis M, Schneider M, et al. Motorised spiral enteroscopy: first prospective clinical feasibility study. Gut. 2021;70:261–7.
31. Beyna T, Arvanitakis M, Schneider M, et al. Total motorized spiral enteroscopy: first prospective clinical feasibility trial. Gastrointest Endosc. 2021;93:1362–70.
32. Rughwani H, Singh AP, Ramchandani M, et al. A randomized, controlled trial comparing the total enteroscopy rate and diagnostic efficacy of novel motorized spiral enteroscopy and single-balloon enteroscopy in patients with small-bowel disorders: the motor trial (NCT 05548140). Am J Gastroenterol. 2023;118:1855–63.
33. Akerman PA, Haniff M. Spiral enteroscopy: prime time or for the happy few? Best Pract Res Clin Gastroenterol. 2012;26:293–301.
34. Judah JR, Draganov PV, Lam Y, Hou W, Buscaglia JM. Spiral enteroscopy is safe and effective for an elderly United States population of patients with numerous comorbidities. Clin Gastroenterol Hepatol. 2010;8:572–6.
35. Prasad M, Prasad VGM, Sangameswaran A, et al. A spiraling journey into the small bowel: a case series of novel motorized power spiral enteroscopies. VideoGIE. 2020;5:591–6.

Atlas of Small Bowel Diseases Diagnosed by Balloon-Assisted Enteroscopy

7

Sung Noh Hong

7.1 Neoplastic Lesions

7.1.1 Small-Bowel Cancer [1]

① Small-bowel adenoma

(A) Isp-type 3-mm jejunal adenoma
(B) Isp-type 3-cm adenoma with high-grade adenoma in the fourth portion of the duodenum causing intussusception
(C), (D) Multiple small-bowel adenomas in a patient with Lynch syndrome
(E) IIa-type 1-cm flat raised adenoma in the jejunum in a patient with familial adenomatous polyposis
(F) Adenomatous lesion clearly delineated by chromoendoscopy with indigo carmine.

S. N. Hong (✉)
Sungkyunkwan University School of Medicine, Seoul, South Korea
e-mail: sungnoh.hong@samsung.com

J.-J. Park et al. (eds.), *Balloon-Assisted Enteroscopy*,
https://doi.org/10.1007/978-981-95-2445-7_7

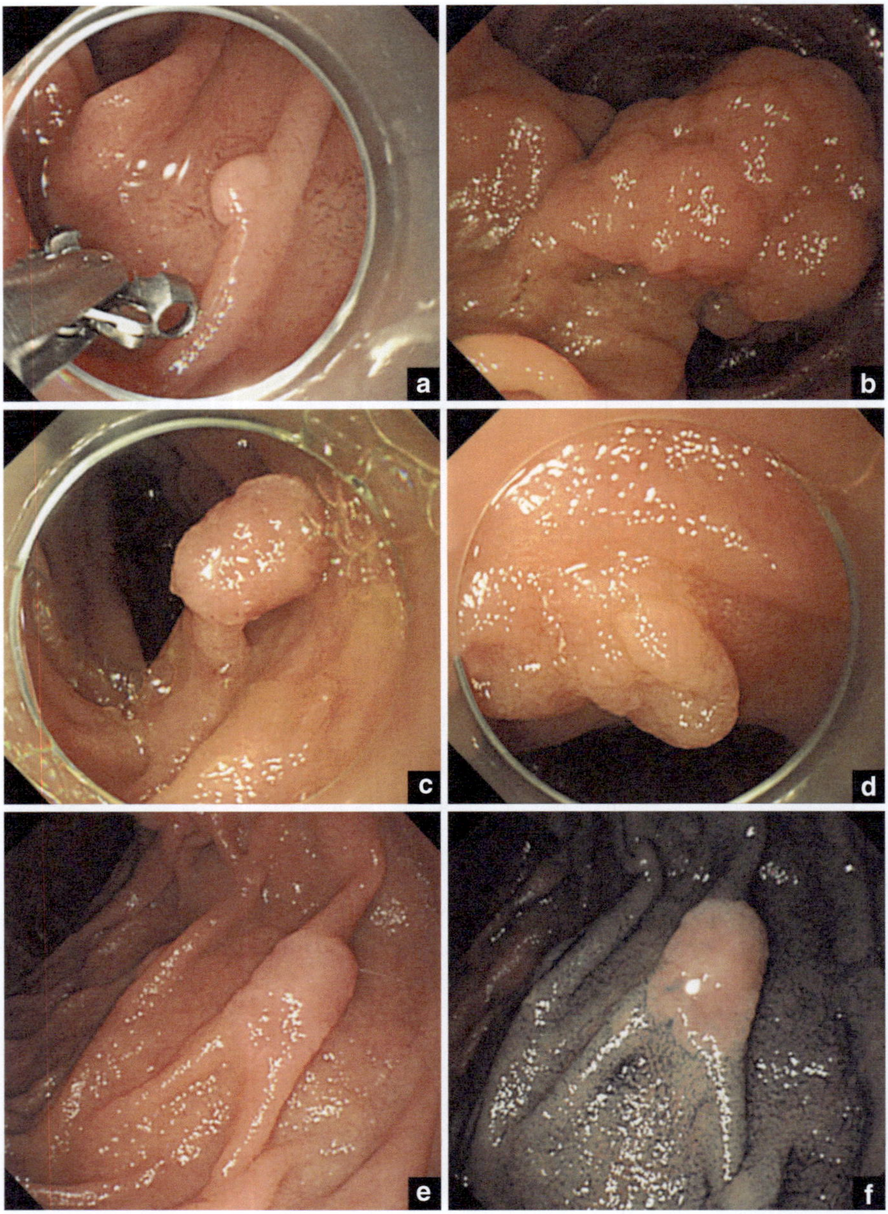

② **Small-bowel adenocarcinoma**

(A) Small-bowel adenocarcinoma with irregularly raised margins and central depression with ulceration in the fourth portion of the duodenum
(B) Jejunal adenocarcinoma with nodular borders and central depression
(C) Small-bowel adenocarcinoma of the protruding type with a nodular surface
(D) Infiltrative-type, flat elevated small-bowel adenocarcinoma

(E) Diffuse infiltrative-type small-bowel adenocarcinoma with luminal narrowing
(F) Ulceroinfiltrative-type small-bowel adenocarcinoma with luminal narrowing
(G) Ulcerofungating-type small-bowel adenocarcinoma with stricture and food stasis
(H) Small-bowel adenocarcinoma of the ulcerative type in a patient with Lynch syndrome.

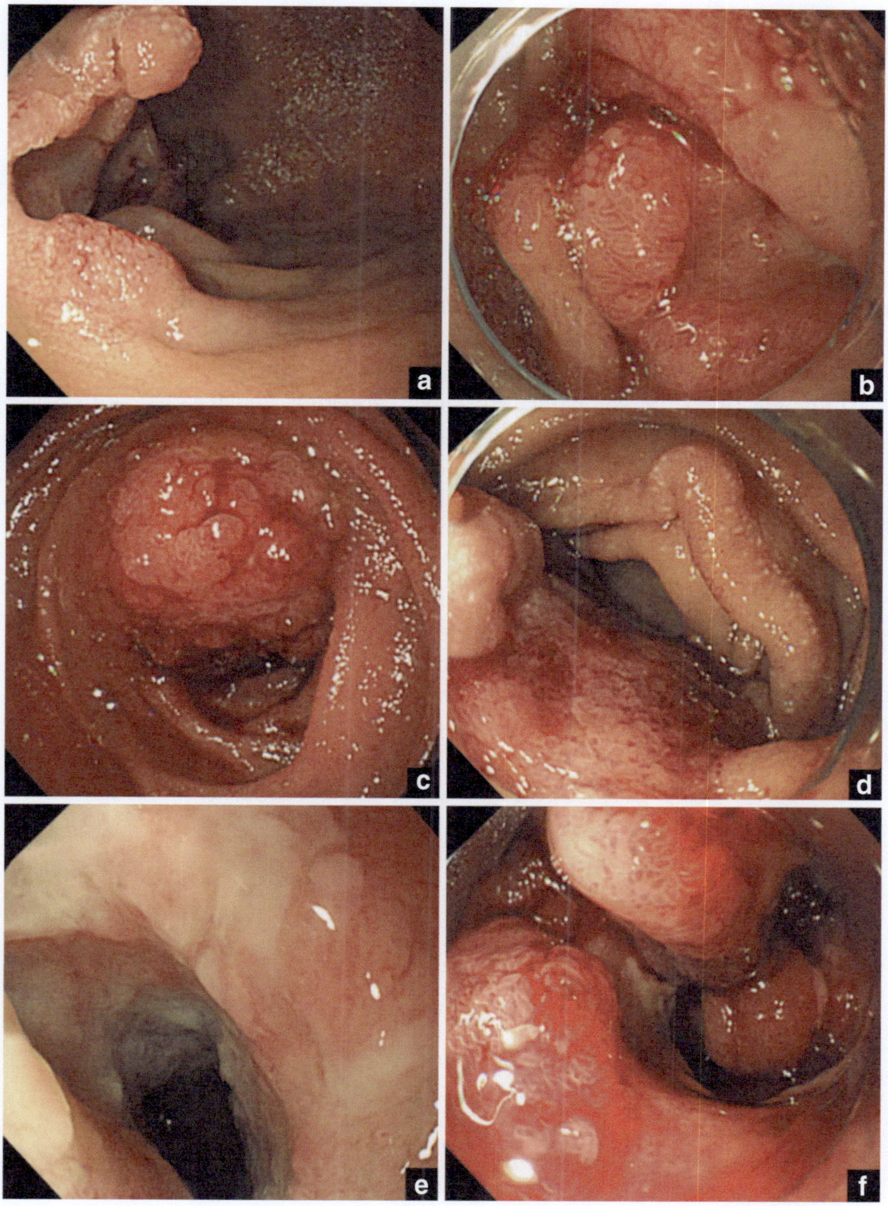

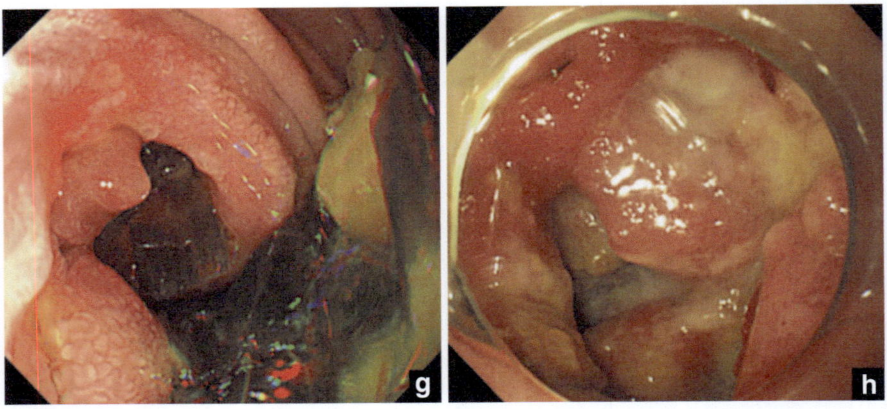

* Tips for diagnosis: Similar to adenocarcinomas identified on the gastrointestinal tracts with conventional endoscopy, advanced-stage small-bowel adenocarcinomas can present as protruding, ulcerative, ulceroinfiltrative, and diffuse infiltrative-type endoscopically on balloon-assisted enteroscopy. Small-bowel adenocarcinoma often present with obstructive symptoms and passage disturbance caused by luminal narrowing.

7.1.2 Lymphoma

① Diffuse large B-cell lymphoma

(A) Mass-like DLBL with a raised margin and central depression in the proximal ileum
(B) Circumferential ileal DLBL with a nodular friable surface
(C) Geographic ulceroinfiltrative DLBL covered with exudates
(D) Nodular-type DLBL mimicking submucosal tumors of variable size with superficial aphthous ulcers in the terminal ileum.

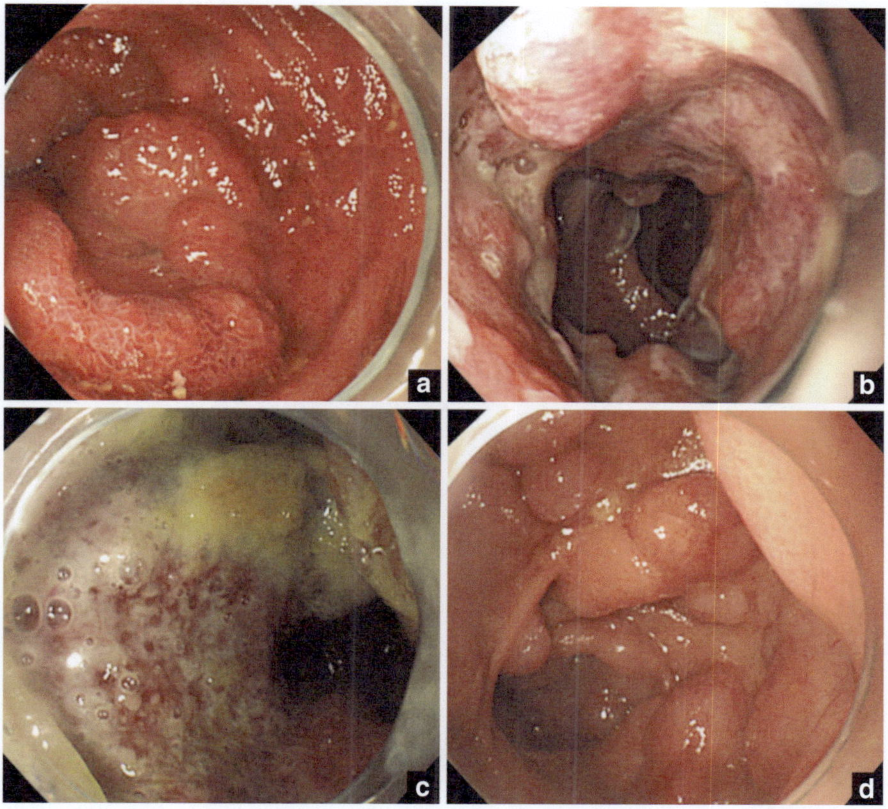

② **Mucosa-assisted lymphoid tissue (MALT) lymphoma**

(A) Low-grade MALT lymphoma with a thickened mucosa and small nodules with indistinct borders

(B) Low-grade MALT lymphoma with patchy depression of discolored infiltration with indistinct borders.

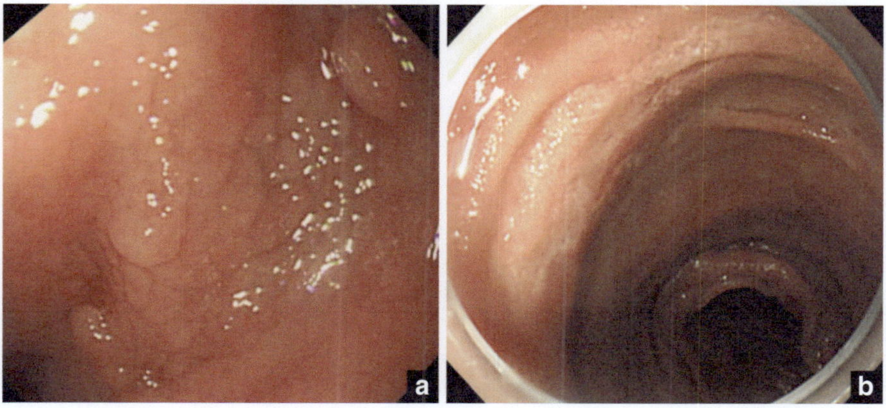

③ Mantle cell lymphoma.

Diffuse infiltrative lesion with erythematous nodular mucosal changes and superficial irregular ulcers in the terminal ileum.

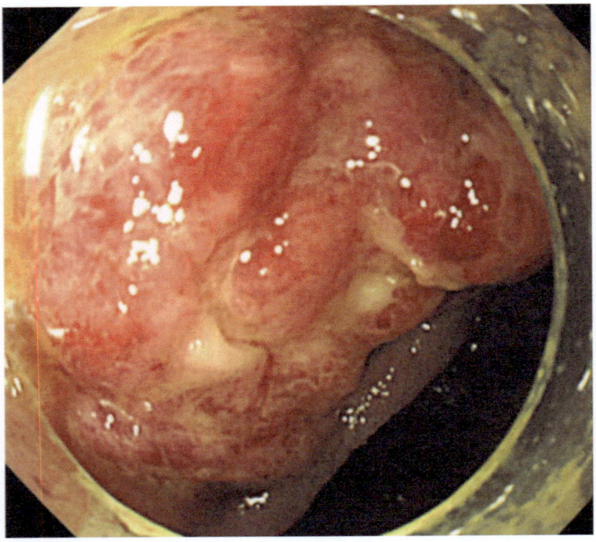

④ Natural killer (NK)/T-cell lymphoma

(A) Large geographic ulcerative lesions with an irregular base and clearly demarcated margin

(B) Multiple geographic ulcers in the jejunum surrounded by inhomogeneous regenerative epithelium and abnormal converging folds.

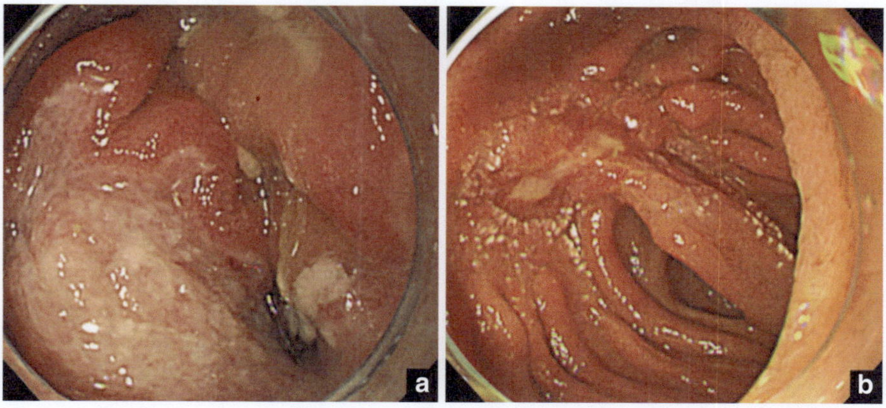

⑤ **Peripheral T-cell lymphoma**

(A) Luminal encircling ulceroinfiltrative lesion with a whitish exudate covering an irregular base in the jejunum

(B) Segmental ulceroinfiltrative lesion with a nodular elevated margin and irregular base identified in multiple parts of the small bowel.

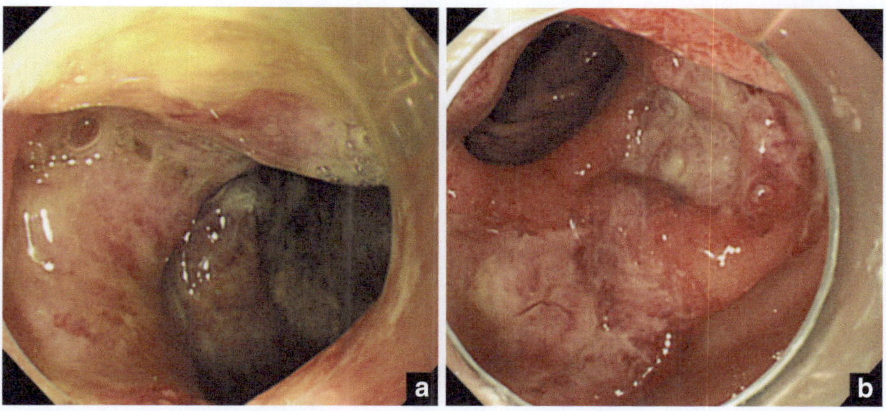

⑥ **Burkitt lymphoma**

Luminal encircling ulceroinfiltrative mass with dirty and thick exudates covering an irregular base in the ileum.

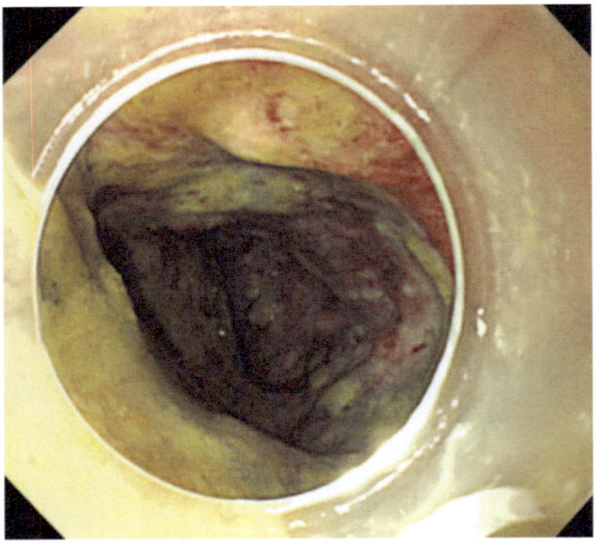

⑦ **Enteropathy-associated T-cell lymphoma** [2]

(A) Diffuse infiltrative lesions with indistinct margins covered by whitish granular and erythematous superficial changes

(B) Atypical superficial ulcerative mass with an irregular base and indistinct margin.

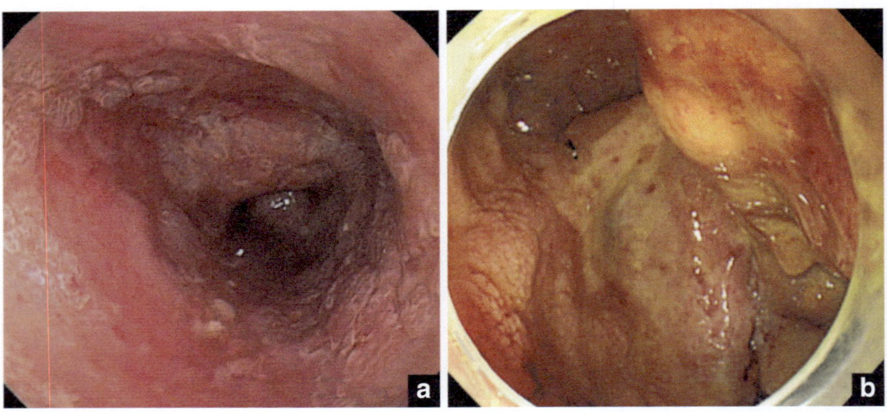

* Tips for diagnosis: Lymphomas have different findings, based on histologic types and origin (from subepithelial lymphoid tissues and lymphocytes), on balloon-assisted enteroscopy. Small bowel tumors often present with nonspecific symptoms such as abdominal pain, weight loss, gastrointestinal bleeding, bowel obstruction, or perforation. Intestinal obstruction is common in small bowel adenocarcinoma, whereas perforation is more common in lymphoma.

7.1.3 Gastrointestinal Stromal Tumor (GIST)

(A) A 1.5-cm jejunal GIST with features of a subepithelial tumor that include a bridging fold overlying the normal mucosa
(B) A 3-cm round mass overlying the normal mucosa with a small central ulcer
(C) A 3-cm round oval subepithelial tumor covered by the normal mucosa in a patient with small-bowel bleeding
(D) An exposed vessel in the umbilication on the surface of this lesion
(E) GIST with a hematoma attached on the central ulcer, indicating recent hemorrhage
(F) Malignant GIST with a deeply depressed ulcer and irregular nodular base.

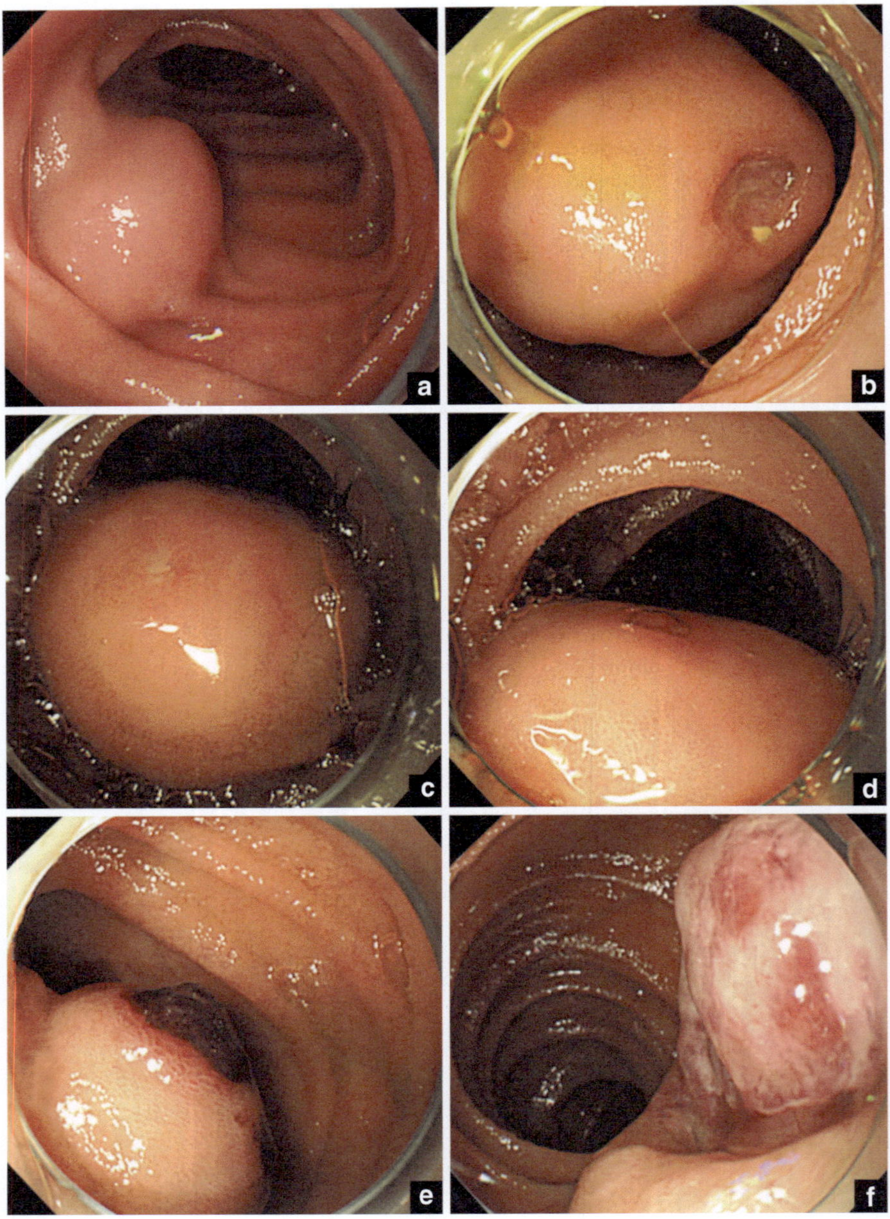

* Tip for diagnosis: Small-bowel GISTs present as round and oval subepithelial tumors with an overlying normal mucosa and bridging folds. Malignant transformation should be considered if a GIST $\geq$2 cm accompanied by umbilication, ulcer, and nodular surface. GIST with central ulcer or umbilication is associated with a risk of bleeding. Considering the subepithelial origin of GIST, unnecessary biopsy should be avoided due to the risk of bleeding.

7.1.4 Neuroendocrine Tumor (NET)

(A) An irregular nodular subepithelial tumor with bridging folds in the fourth portion of the duodenum
(B) A small, flat elevated yellowish polypoid subepithelial tumor with superficial erythematous changes in the fourth part of the duodenum
(C) A malignant NET with elevated margins, irregularly shaped central depressions, and nodular surface in the third portion of the duodenum
(D) A malignant NET with luminal semi-encircling ulcerative infiltrative lesion in the second portion of the duodenum. The base of the depressed lesion was irregular and had a nodular surface with hyperemia and telangiectasia.

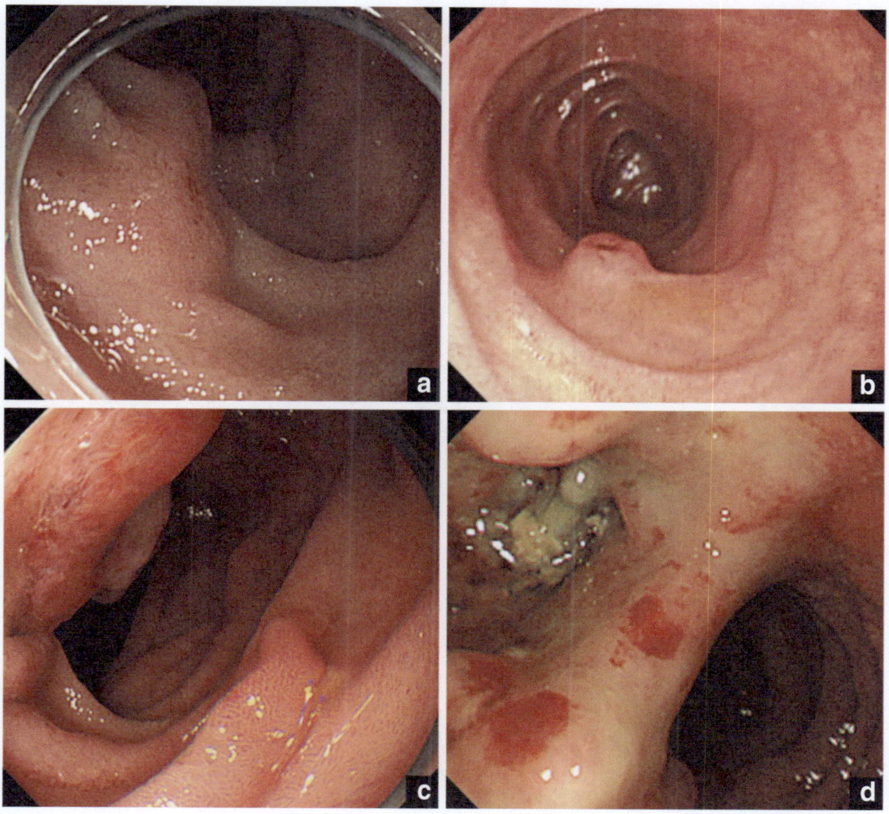

7.1.5 Metastatic Cancer

(A) Metastatic lung cancer: An ulceroinfiltrative mass with a friable mucosal margin and whitish thick exudates covering the jejunum
(B) Metastatic lung cancer: An irregular and nodular circumferential protruding mass with superficial ulcer at the border of the jejunum and the ileum
(C) Metastatic lung cancer: An infiltrative luminal protruding mass with a central ulcer with an irregular border and friable mucosa in the ileum
(D) Metastatic liposarcoma: A subepithelial tumor-like protruding mass with a central deep ulcer and infiltrative friable margin in the duodenum.

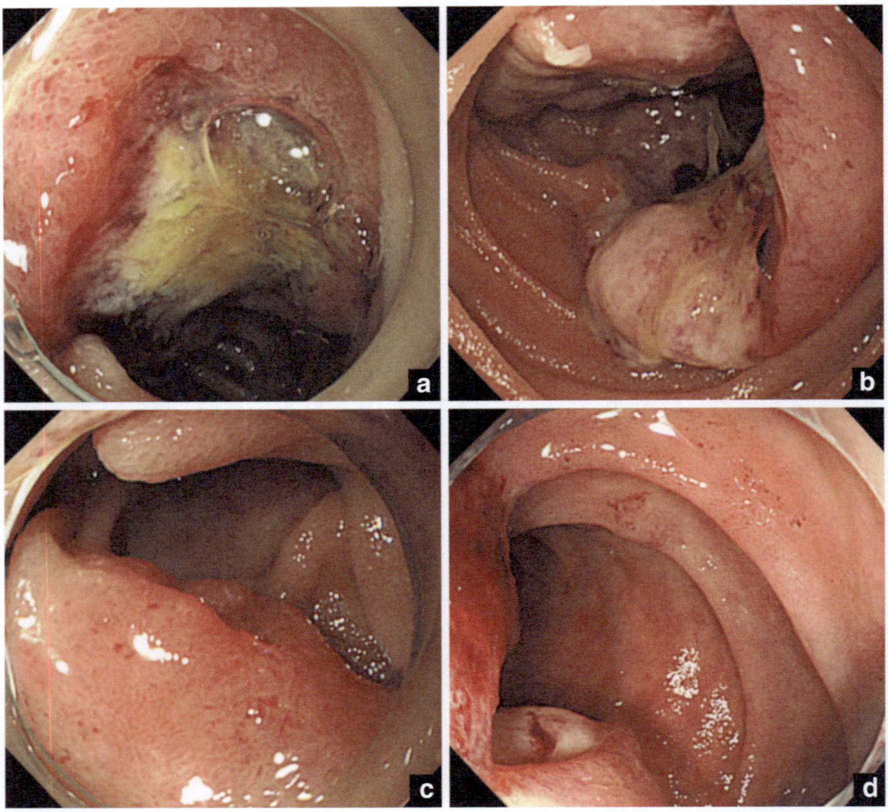

7.1.6 Hamartomatous Polyps of Peutz-Jeghers Syndrome [3]

(A) Multiple hamartomatous polyps on the jejunum in a patient with Peutz-Jeghers syndrome
(B) Isp-type 8-mm jejunal hamartomatous polyps in a patient with Peutz-Jeghers syndrome
(C) Isp-type 12-mm ileal hamartomatous polyps in a patient with Peutz-Jeghers syndrome

(D) Isp-type 20-mm jejunal hamartomatous polyps in a patient with Peutz-Jeghers syndrome

(E), (F) Endoscopic mucosal resection for Isp-type 15-mm jejunal hamartomatous polyps in a patient with Peutz-Jeghers syndrome.

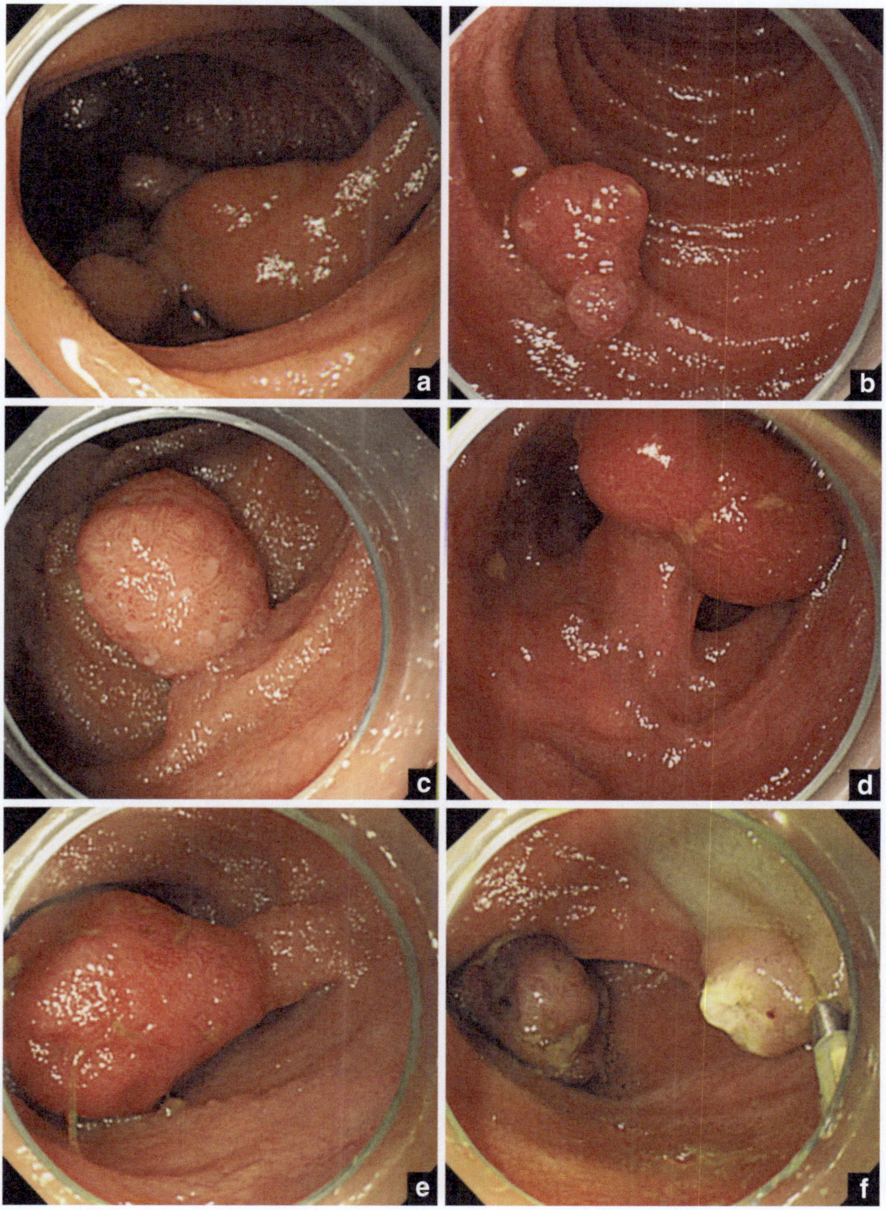

7.1.7 Hemangioma

(A) Proximal jejunal capillary hemangioma measuring 8 mm with superficial punctate dilated capillaries, (B) intermittent bleeding
(C) Cavernous hemangioma with a bluish nodular protruding mass measuring 15 mm on the jejunum and a dilated vascular structure on the surface of the lesion
(D) Cavernous hemangioma with a 2-cm Isp-shaped, polypoid, bluish nodular protruding mass with superficial erythema in the fourth portion of the duodenum.

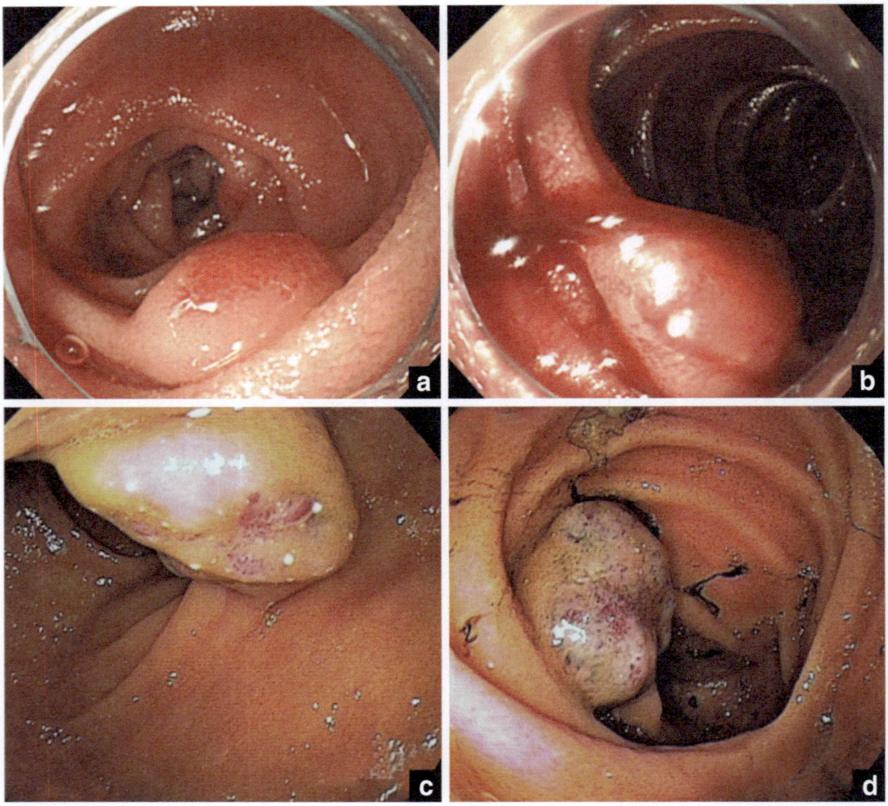

7.1.8 Ectopic Pancreas

(A) Slightly elevated white-yellowish and infiltrative lesion with indistinct borders in the proximal jejunum. A small, depressed structure suspected to be a pancreatic duct orifice
(B) Slightly elevated infiltrative lesion with a nodular surface with indistinct borders in the proximal jejunum and a central depression suspected to be a pancreatic duct opening

(C) Slightly elevated infiltrative lesion with indistinct borders in the fourth part of the duodenum
(D) Isp-type nodular whitish-yellowish protruding subepithelial lesion with an overlying normal mucosa in the proximal jejunum.

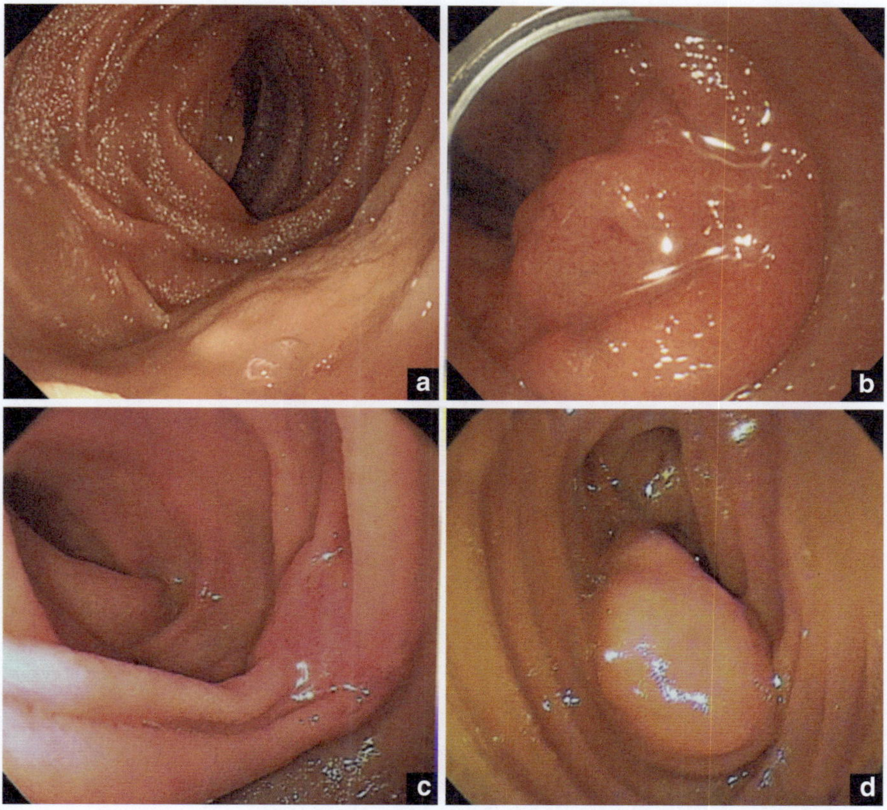

7.1.9 Lipoma

(A) A 1.5-cm yellowish Isp-type subepithelial tumor in the ileum that was soft and compressible when pressed with biopsy forceps (positive pillow sign)
(B) A 2-cm Isp-type subepithelial tumor in the jejunum that was soft and compressible when pressed with biopsy forceps (positive pillow sign).
(C) A large lipoma with superficial ulceration caused by recurrent transient intussusception in the proximal jejunum, filling almost the whole lumen of the intestine
(D) Yellow adipose tissues in the resected section after endoscopic mucosal resection (naked fat sign).

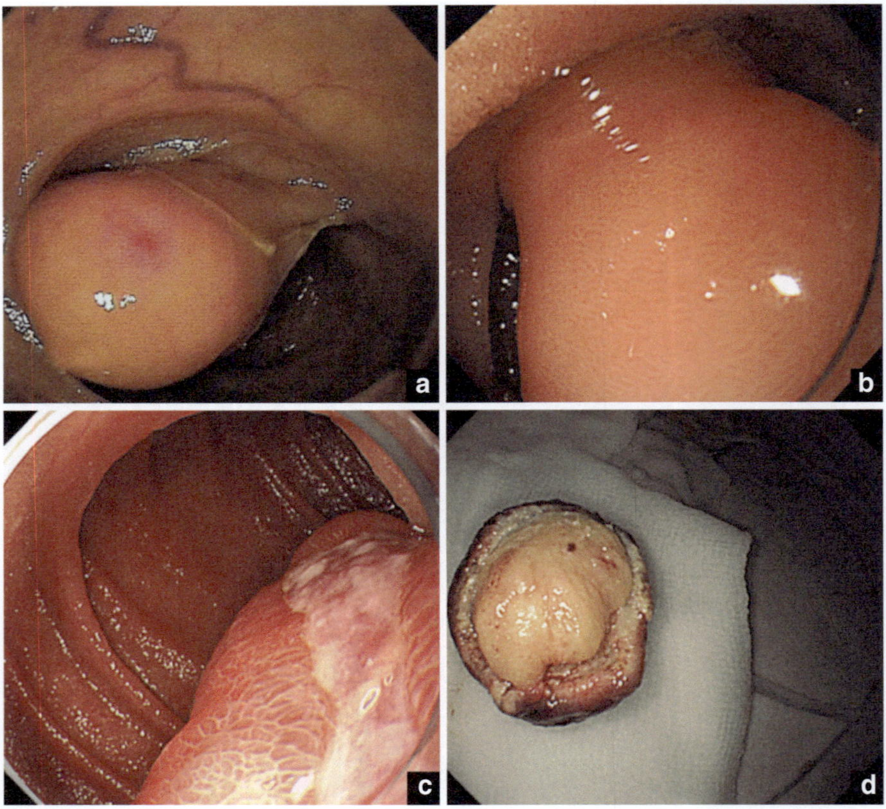

7.2 Inflammatory Lesions

7.2.1 Small-Bowel Crohn's Disease [4, 5]

(A–D) Longitudinal ulcers located asymmetrically at the mesenteric border of the small intestine
(E), (F) Eccentric longitudinal ulcer with shortening of the mesenteric border with luminal narrowing and ulcerative scar and saccular dilatation with antimesenteric border
(G) Longitudinally arranged aphthous ulcers
(H) Cobblestone appearance of the small intestinal mucosa with ulceration
(I–L) Inflammatory stricture with transverse circular ulceration
(M) Web-like fibrotic stricture
(N) Eccentric fibrotic stricture with an eccentric longitudinal ulcer scar
(O), (P) Endoscopic balloon dilation using balloon-assisted enteroscopy for small-bowel stricture in a patient with Crohn's disease.

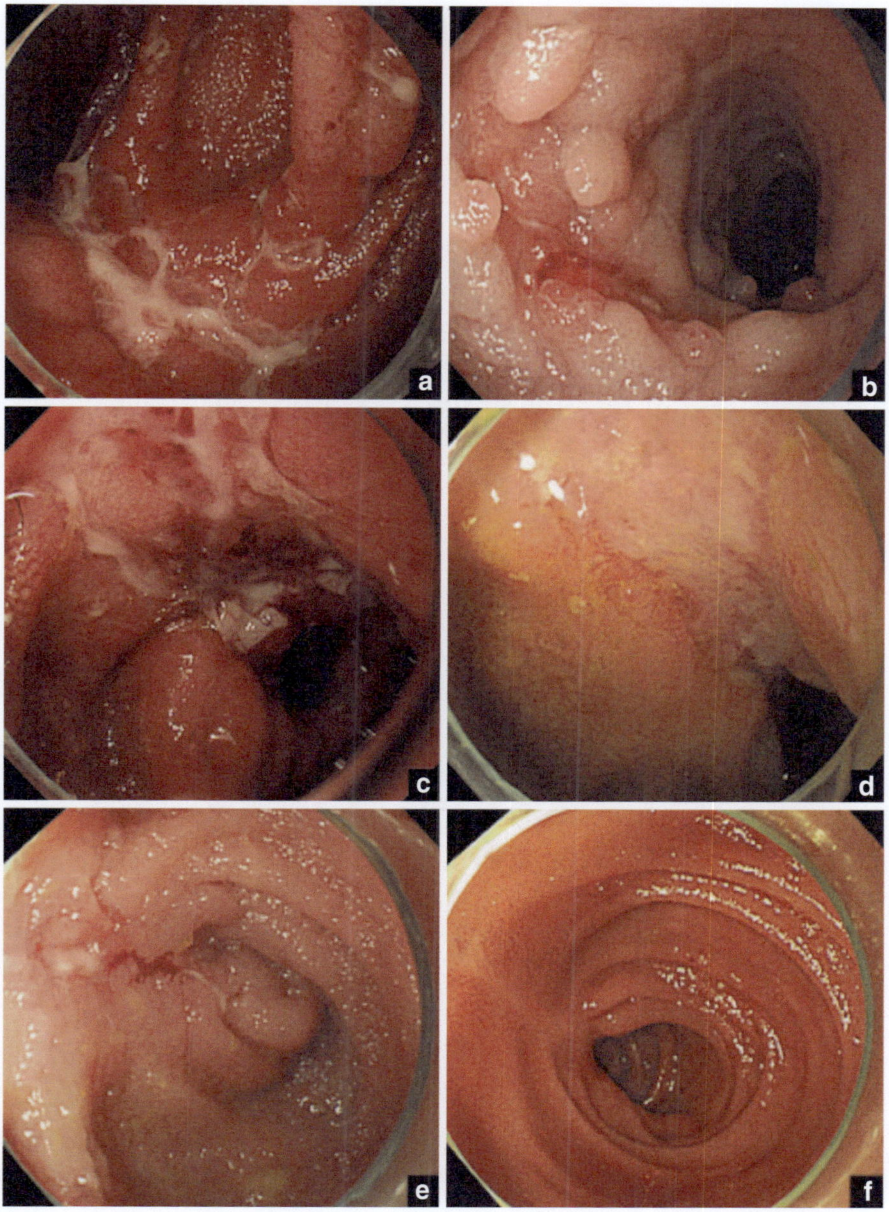
a
b
c
d
e
f

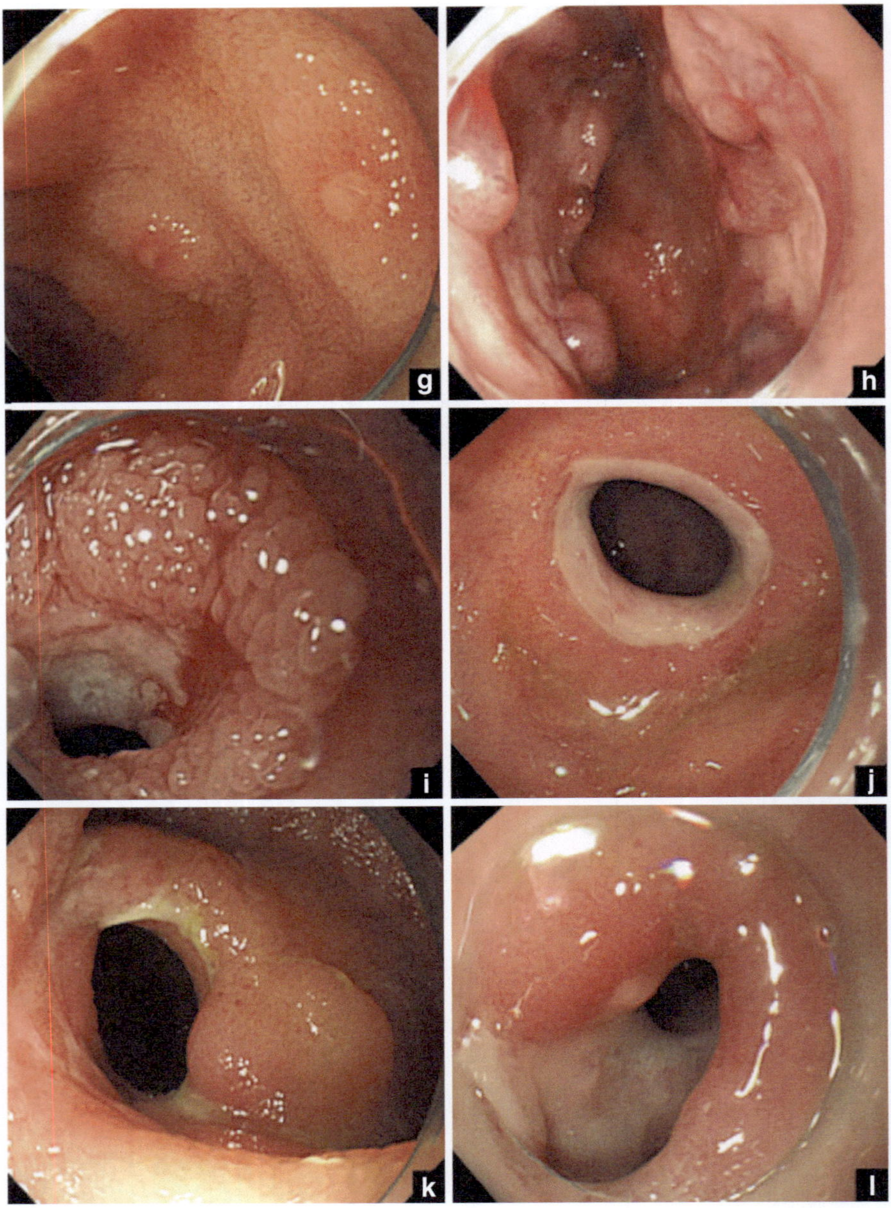
g
h
i
j
k
l

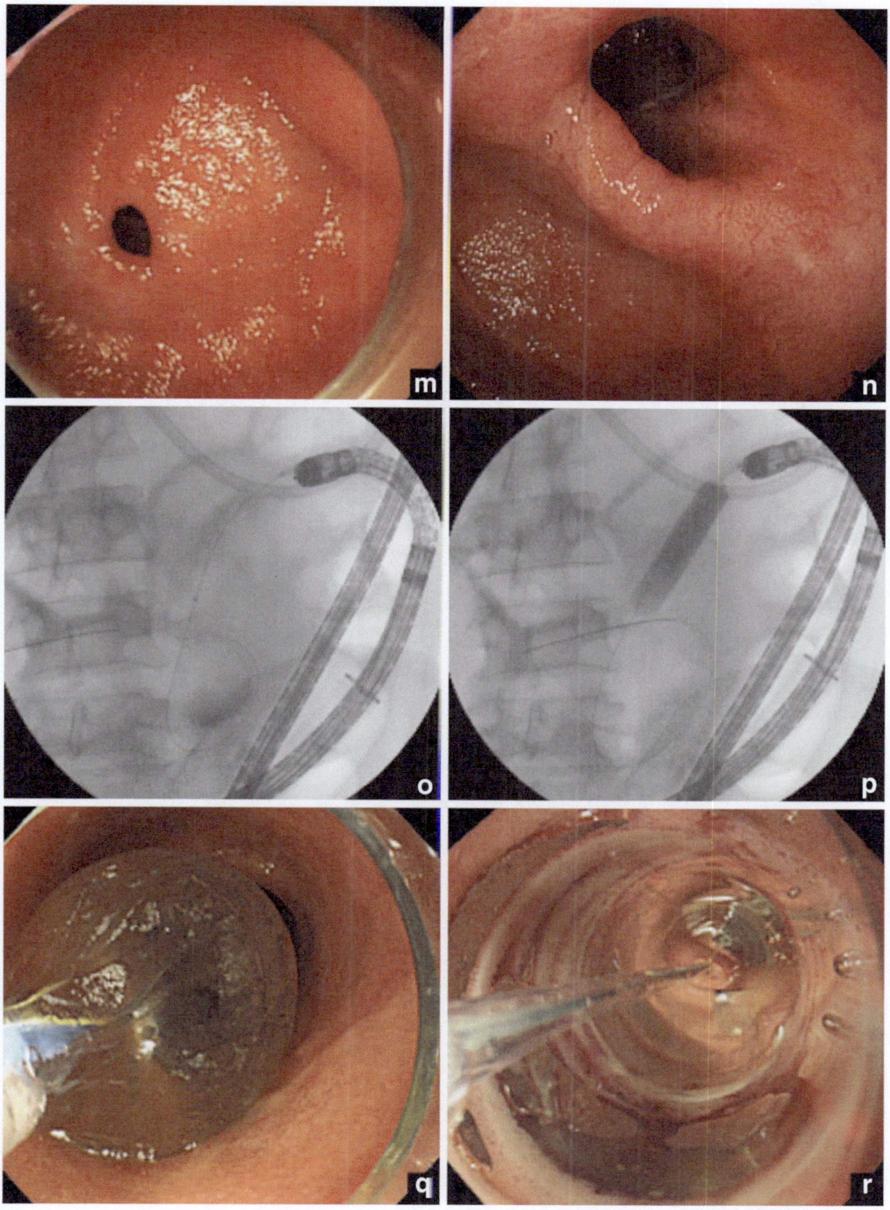

* Tips for diagnosis: On balloon-assisted enteroscopy, small-bowel Crohn's disease is characterized by non-contiguous longitudinal ulcers, longitudinally arranged aphthous ulcers, and a cobblestone appearance. In addition, transverse circular ulcers are often observed, resulting in inflammatory strictures of the small bowel.

7.2.2 Small-Bowel Tuberculosis

(A), (B) Small-bowel tuberculosis identified as segmental ileal strictures with edematous mucosa and ulceration (no evidence of pulmonary tuberculosis; chronic active ileitis with caseating granulomas on histological examination and *Mycobacterium tuberculosis* isolated in the acid-fast bacteria culture)

(C, D) Small-bowel tuberculosis diagnosed in a patient with pulmonary tuberculosis. Luminal narrowing with segmental ulceration in the ileum accompanied by edematous and erythematous mucosal changes.

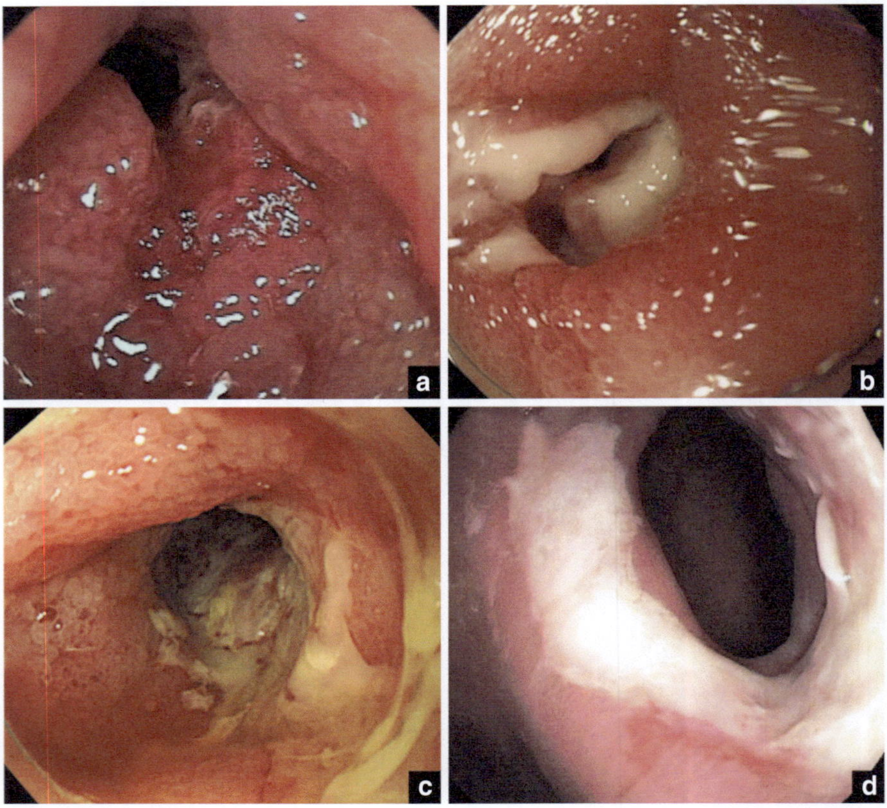

7.2.3 Intestinal Behçet's Disease

(A) Single aphthous ulcers in the terminal ileum of a patient with Behçet's disease

(B) Multiple small aphthous ulcers diffusely distributed in the ileum of a patient with Behçet's disease

(C) Whitish exudates covering a geographically shaped discrete ulcer in the distal ileum of a patient with Behçet's disease

(D) Deep ulcer with a raised margin, folds convergence, and luminal narrowing in the distal ileum of a patient with Behçet's disease.

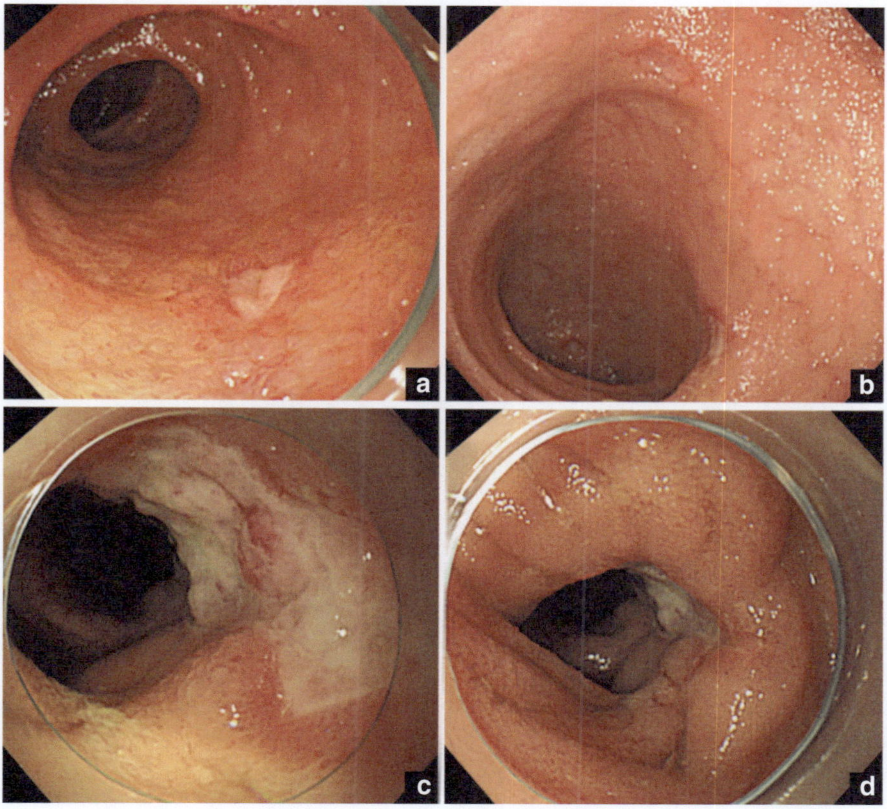

7.2.4 Nonsteroidal Anti-inflammatory Drug (NSAID)-Induced Small-Bowel Ulcer and Enteropathy

(A) Deep discrete ulceration of the distal ileum after the prolonged use of NSAIDs
(B) A healed scar 6 months after the discontinuation of NSAIDs
(C–F) Multiple web-like strictures in the jejunum in a patient with chronic NSAID use
(G), (H) NSAID-induced small-bowel stricture treated with endoscopic balloon dilation using balloon-assisted enteroscopy.

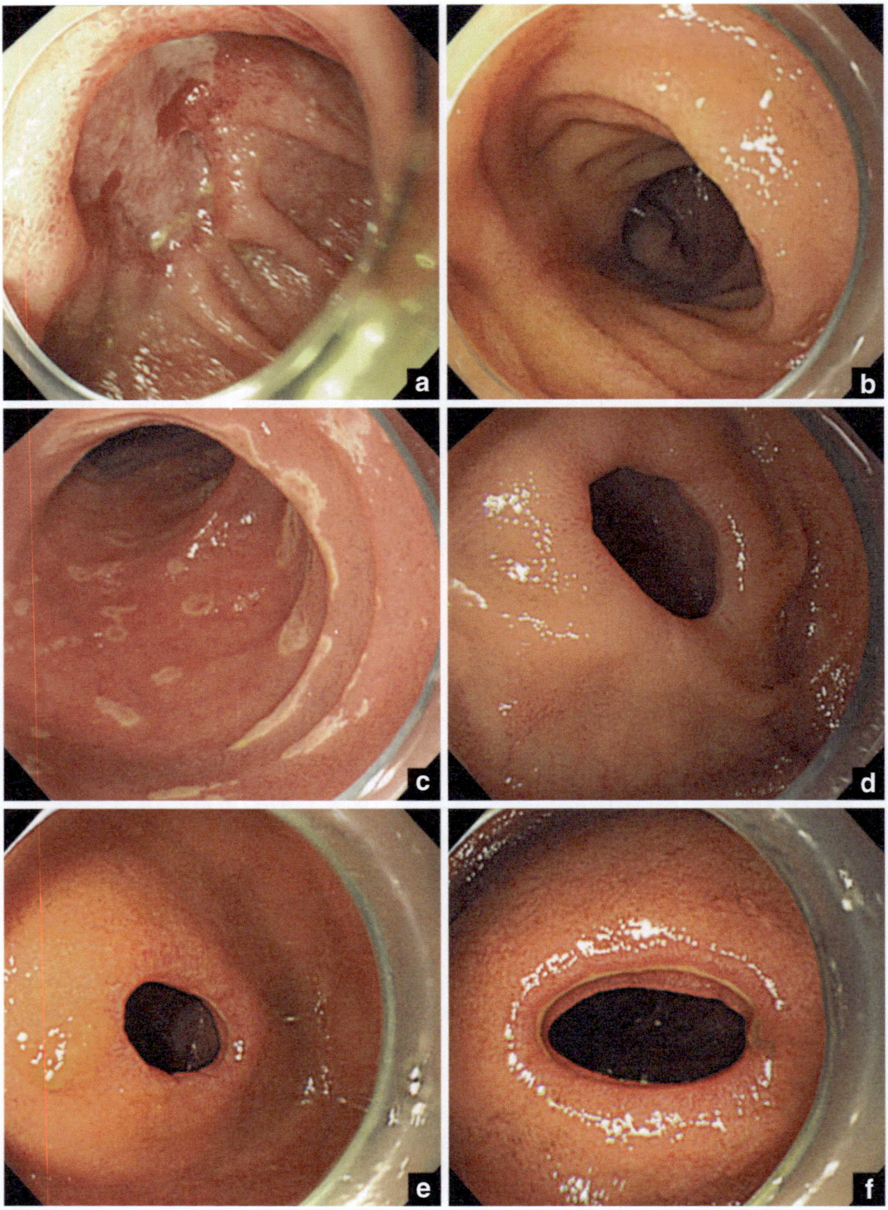
a
b
c
d
e
f

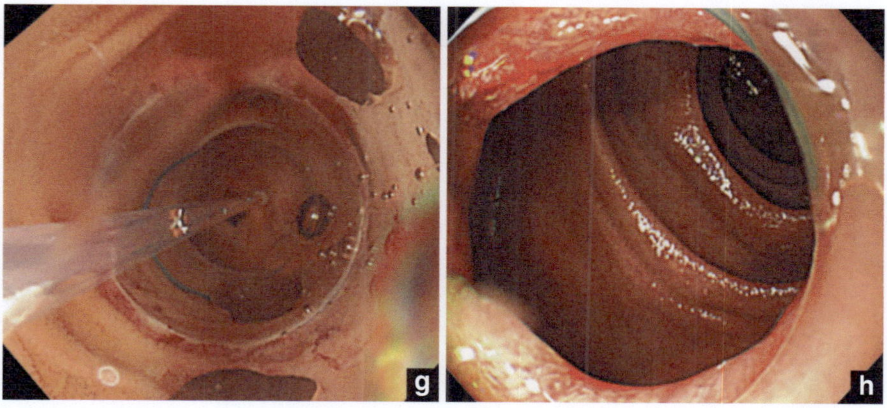

7.2.5 Ischemic Enteritis

(A) Acute ischemic enteritis developed after angiographic embolization for proximal jejunal angioectasia, with a well-demarcated ulcer with necrotic debris clearly demarcated from the normal mucosa
(B), (C) Chronic ischemic enteritis caused by superior mesenteric artery occlusion, with a diffuse well-demarcated superficial ulcer with luminal narrowing and clear demarcation from the normal mucosa
(D) Single-balloon endoscopy after the resolution of the superior mesenteric artery occlusion, showing a large resolved ulcerative lesion of the small intestine.

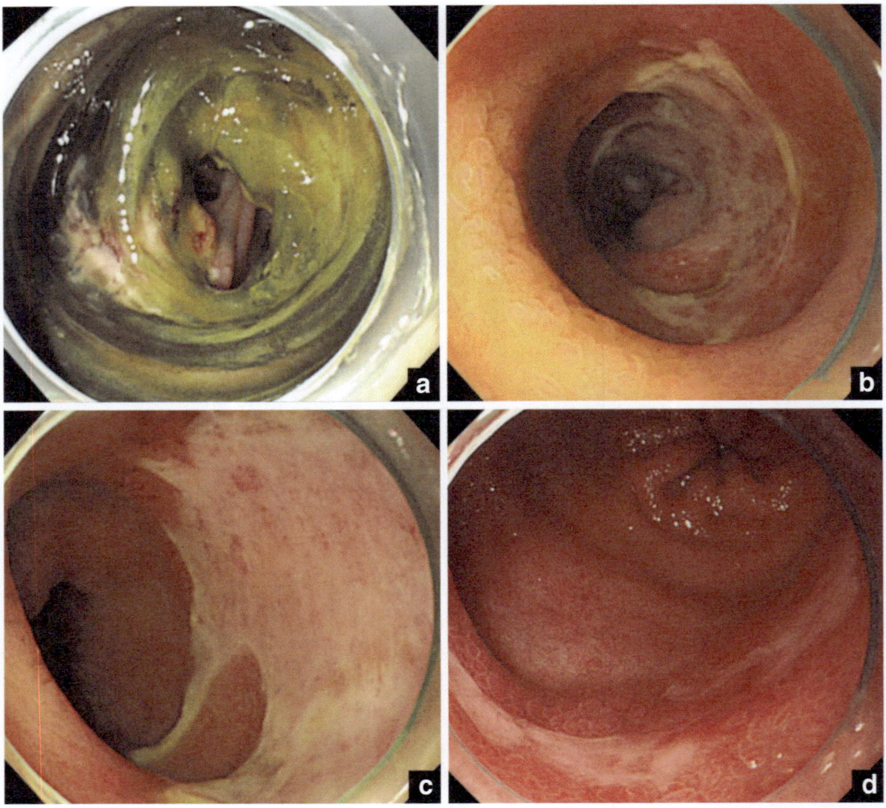

7.2.6 Graft-Versus-Host Disease (GVHD)

(A) Grade 1 GVHD with a patchy distributed edematous mucosa and loss of vasculature
(B) Grade 2 GVHD with diffuse edematous mucosal changes, granularity, and pale exudate
(C) Grade 3 GVHD with marked diffuse edematous mucosal change accompanied by multiple erythema and deep erosions
(D) Grade 4 GVHD with multiple superficial ulcerations covered with whitish exudate and necrotic debris.

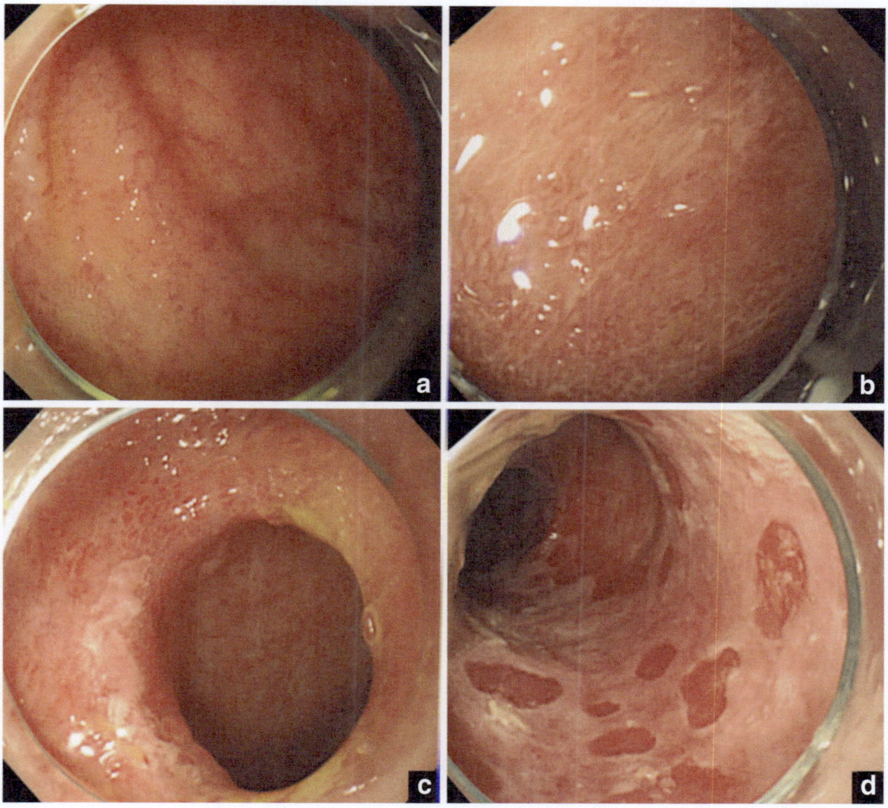

7.2.7 Cytomegalovirus (CMV) Enteritis

(A) Erythematous and edematous mucosal changes in the jejunum of a leukemia patient treated with bone marrow transplantation. Detection of CMV via immunohistochemistry
(B) Shallow well-demarcated ulcerations with exudate in a patient treated with chemotherapy for metastatic colorectal cancer
(C) Geographically shaped ulcerations with an irregular border and base in a patient with glomerulonephritis treated with systemic glucocorticoids (positive CMV immunohistochemistry)
(D) CMV co-infection in ileal ulcers in patients with Crohn's disease (positive CMV immunohistochemistry)
(E) CMV jejunitis in a 64-year-old immunocompetent patient without underlying diseases other than diabetes. Note that the diffuse erythematous and edematous mucosal changes with geographic ulceration with indistinct borders from the proximal to the distal jejunum
(F) CMV ileitis in an 80-year-old immunocompetent patient with well-defined borders and deep ulcerations leading to strictures.

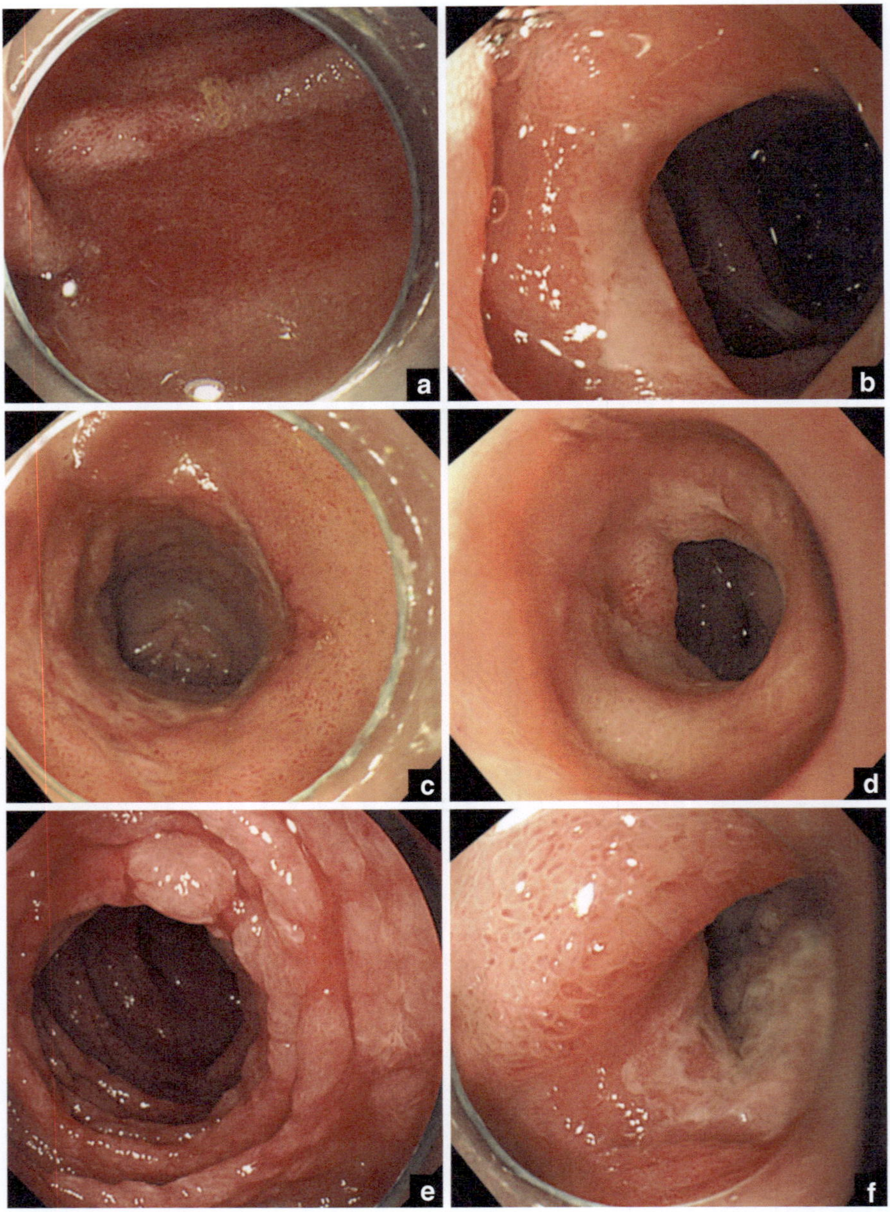
a
b
c
d
e
f

7.2.8 Eosinophilic Enteritis

(A) Edematous and hyperemic mucosal change with granularity and fragility in the ileum (eosinophils 50 per high power field (HPF))
(B) Diffuse edematous mucosal change with mild ulceration (eosinophils 30 per HPF)
(C) Eosinophilic enteritis presented with the presence of swollen, bumpy patches.

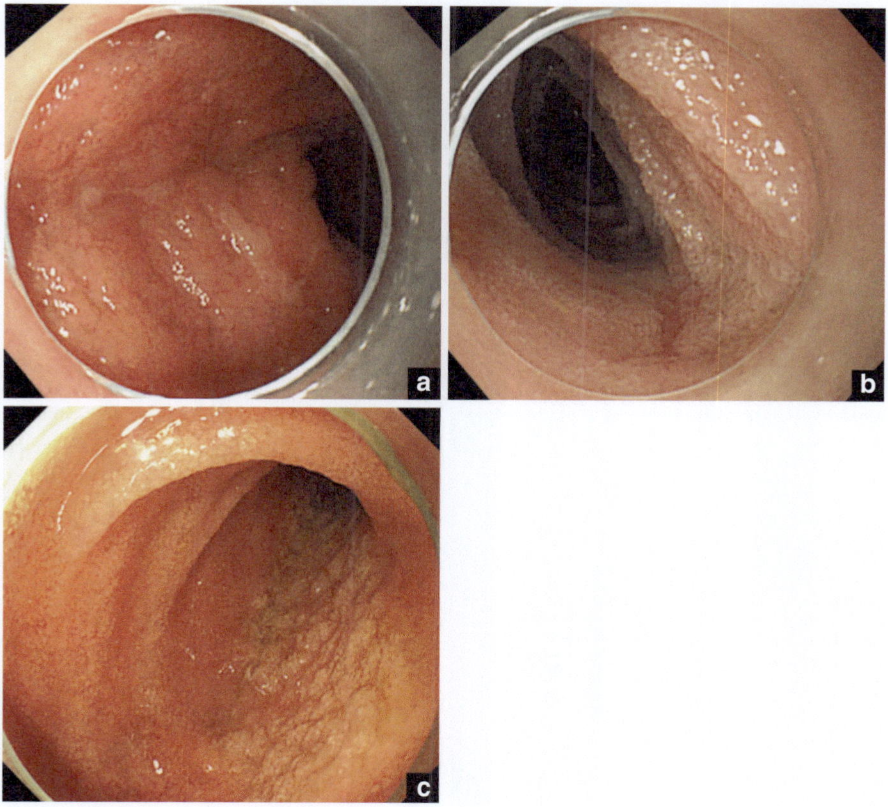

7.2.9 Radiation Enteritis

(A) Acute radiation enteritis with diffuse erythematous and edematous mucosal changes with superficial ulceration after radiotherapy of lymph node metastases in the aortic bifurcation
(B) Chronic radiation enteritis with multiple telangiectasias after radiotherapy for hepatocellular carcinoma.

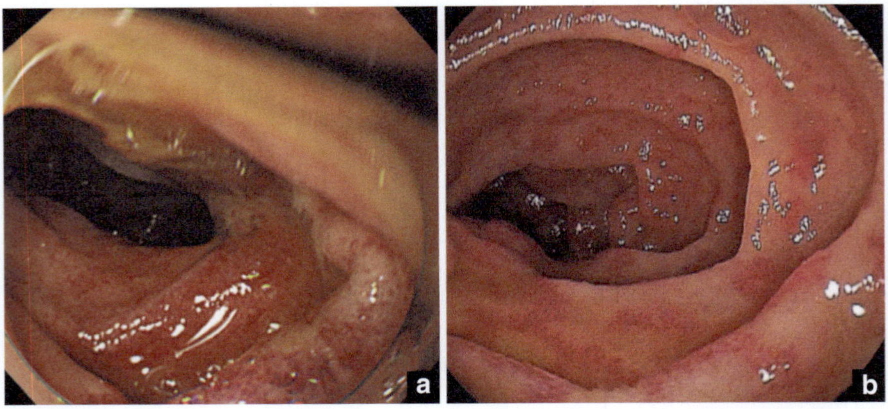

7.2.10 Henoch-Schönlein Purpura

(A), (B) Small bowel involvement in Henoch-Schönlein purpura with multiple well-demarcated edema, severe erythema, and ulceration in the duodenum and the jejunum.

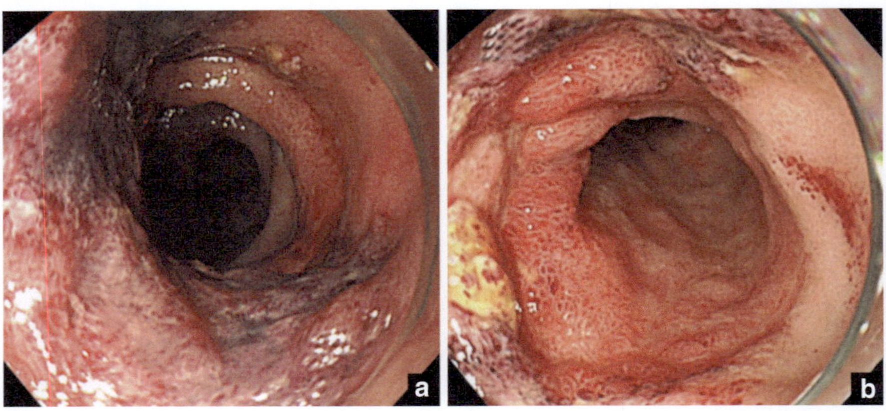

7.3 Small-Bowel Vascular Lesions

7.3.1 Endoscopic Classification of Small-Bowel Vascular Lesion (Yano-Yamamoto Classification) [6]

(A) Yano-Yamamoto type IA small-bowel vascular lesions. Small punctate erythema (< 1 mm), indicating angioectasia

(B–E) Yano-Yamamoto type IB small bowel vascular lesions. Patchy erythema (2–5 mm), indicating a large angioectasia.

(F), (G) Yano-Yamamoto type IIA small bowel vascular lesions. Small punctate lesions (< 1 mm) with active bleeding, indicating Dieulafoy's lesions.

(H), (I) Yano-Yamamoto type IIB small-bowel vascular lesions. Pulsatile red protrusions without surrounding venous dilatation, indicating Dieulafoy's lesions.

(J) Yano-Yamamoto type III small-bowel vascular lesions. Pulsatile red protrusion accompanied by a surrounding venous dilatation, indicating arteriovenous malformations

(K) Yano-Yamamoto type IV small-bowel vascular lesions. An unclassified vascular lesion that does not fit into the other categories.

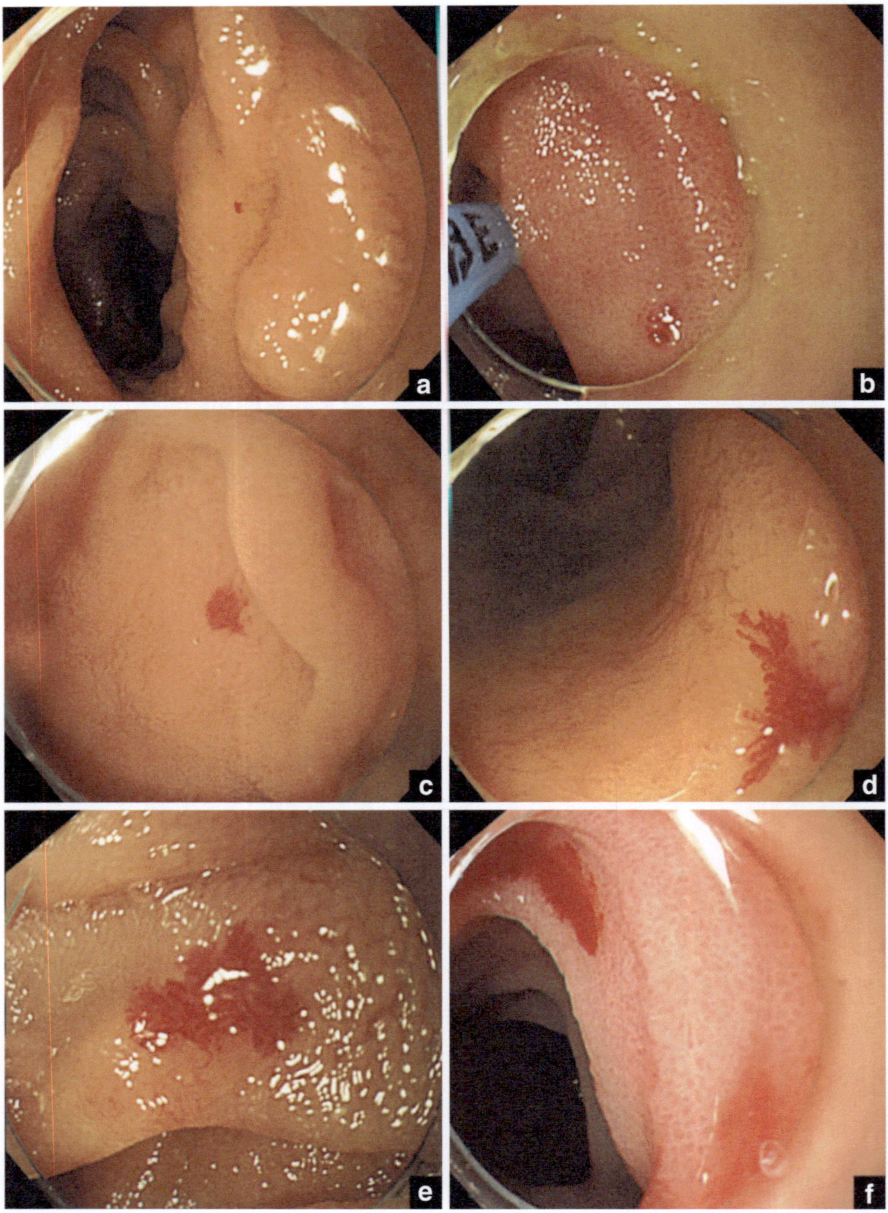
a
b
c
d
e
f

7.3.2 Lymphangiectasia

(A), (B) Whitish dilated lymphangiectasia measuring approximately 5 mm in the proximal jejunum

(C–E) Diffusely distributed whitish dilated lymphangiectasia in the duodenum and the jejunum in a patient with lymphangiectasia leading to protein-losing enteropathy

(F) Lymphangiectasia associated with angioectasia.

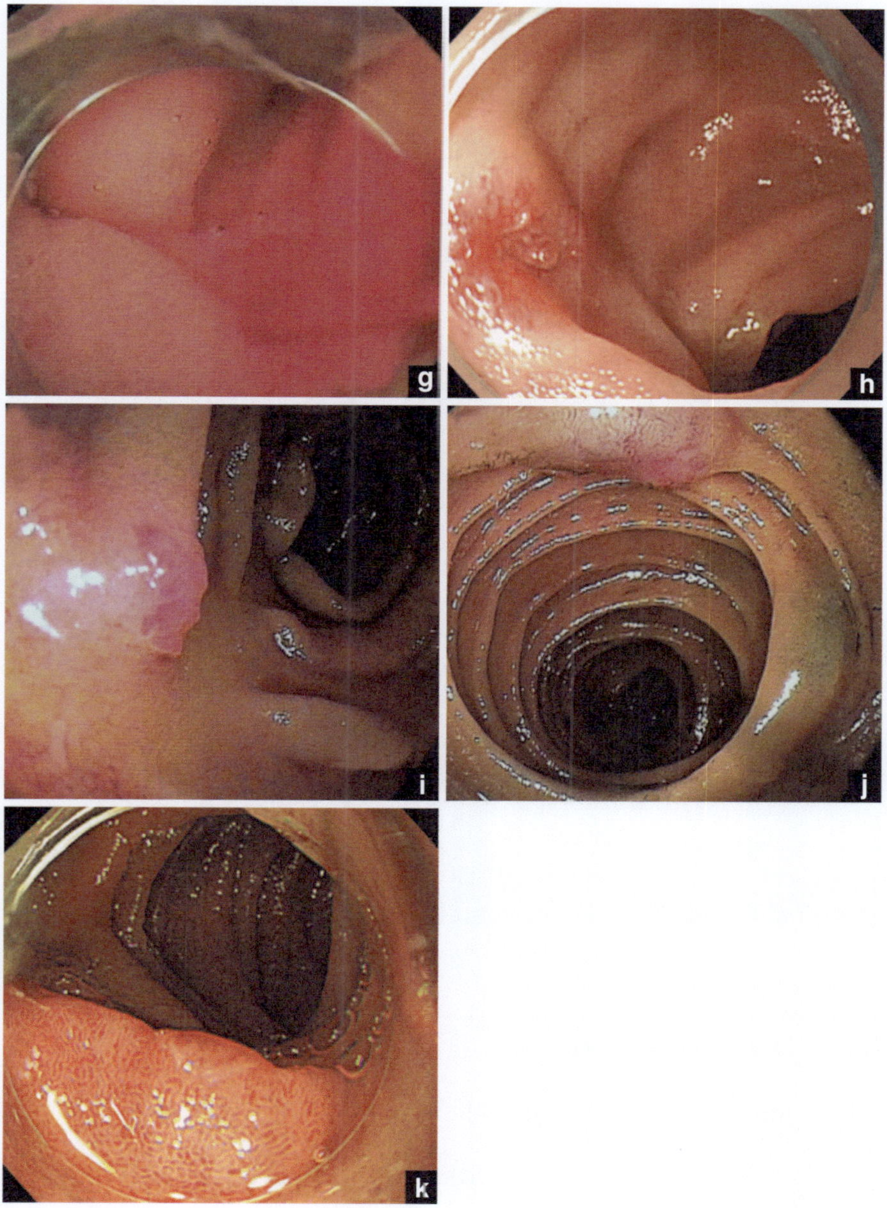

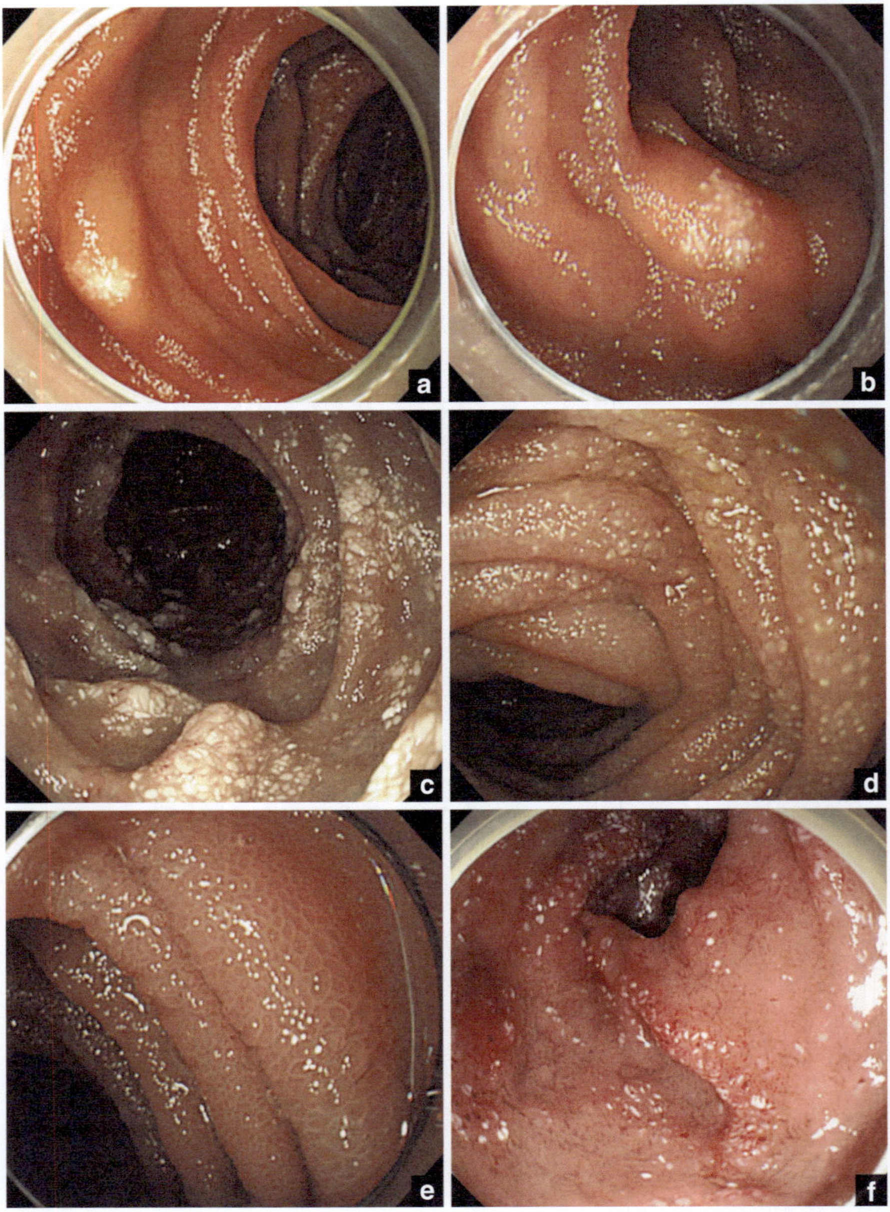

7.4 Diverticular Lesions

7.4.1 Meckel's Diverticulum [7]

(A–C) Two-lumen sign appearing to divide the ileum into two at 100 cm from the ileocecal valve, indicating Meckel's diverticulum.

(D–F) Ulceration in the ectopic gastric tissue in the Meckel's diverticulum.

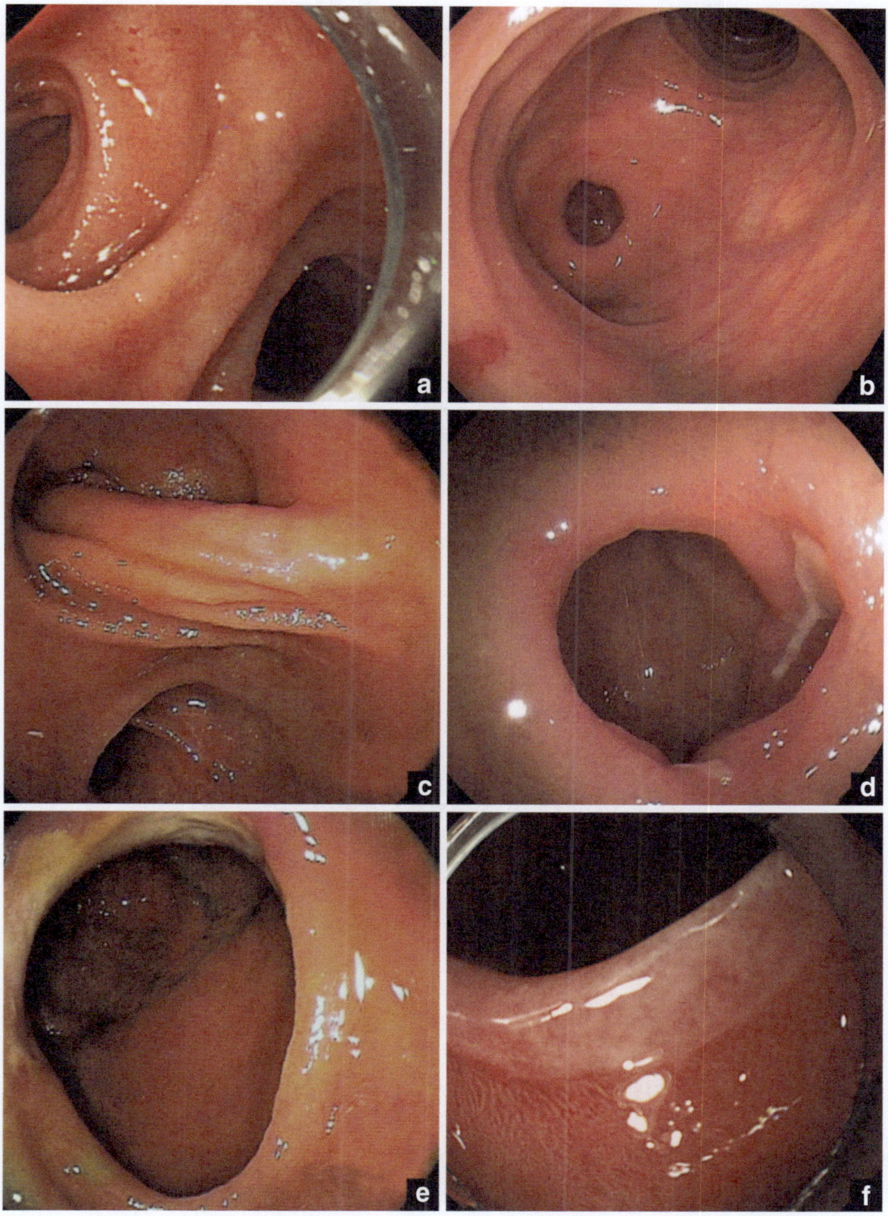

7.4.2 Small-Bowel Diverticulum

(A), (B) Luminal out-pouching diverticulum in the second duodenal portion around the ampulla of Vater
(C), (D) Luminal out-pouching diverticulum in the proximal ileum.

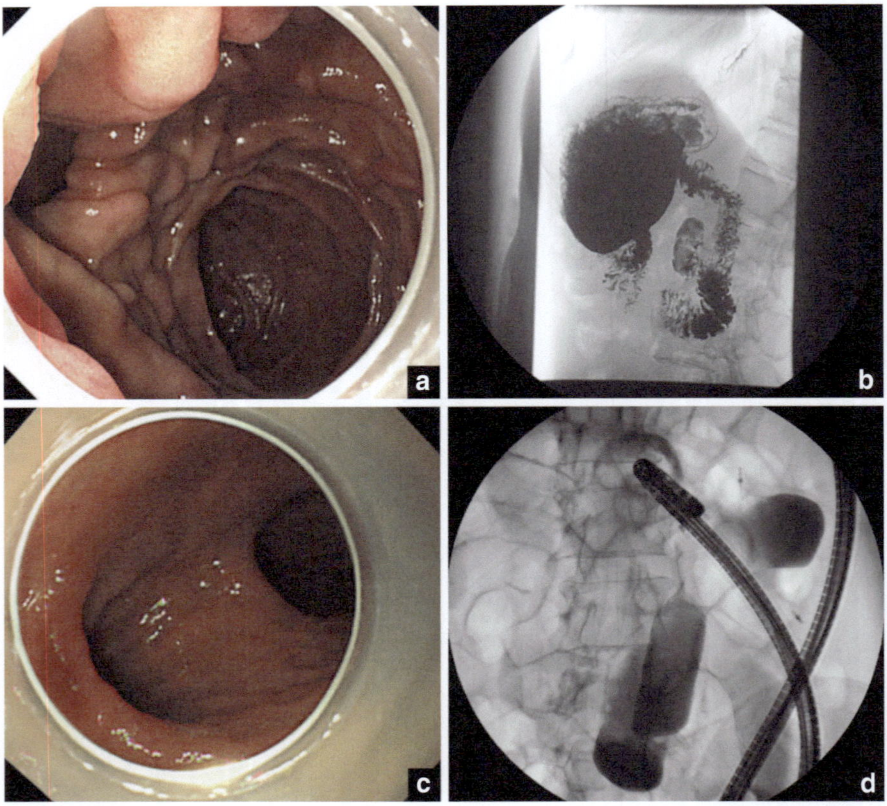

7.5 Miscellaneous Small-Bowel Disease

7.5.1 Amyloidosis

(A) (B) Atypical diffuse edematous and hyperemic mucosal changes with fragility and infiltration with an irregularly shaped material
(C) Luminal narrowing with edematous mucosa with hypertrophied villi in the jejunum.

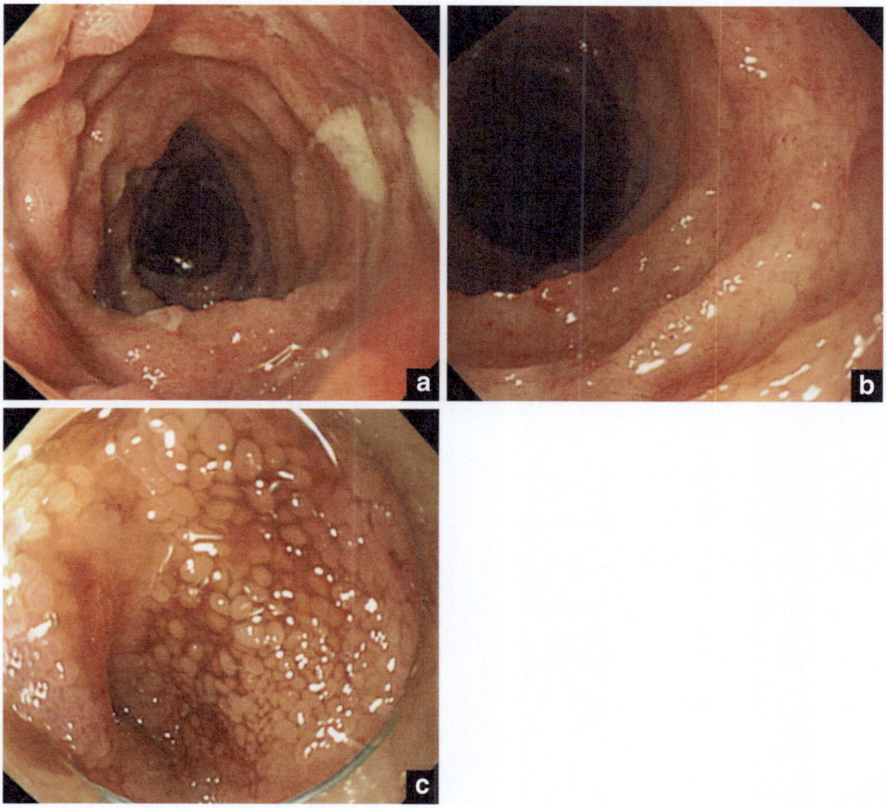

7.5.2 Foreign Body in the Small Bowel

(A–D) Retention of the capsule endoscope at the site of jejunal stricture in a patient with Crohn's disease. Endoscopic balloon dilation was performed, and the capsule endoscope was retrieved with a snare

(E–G) Removal of a displaced esophageal stent in the proximal jejunum.

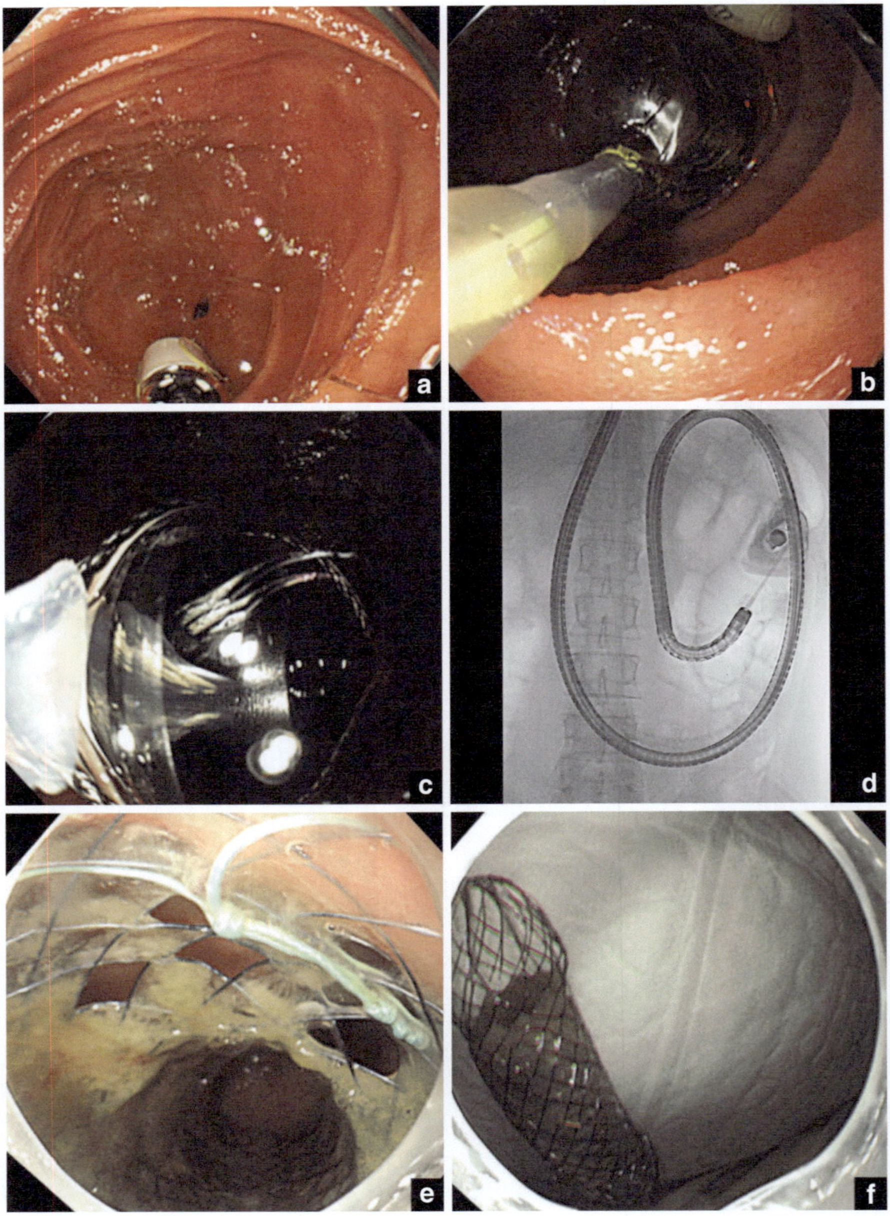
a
b
c
d
e
f

7.5.3 Intestinal Adhesion

(A), (B) Intestinal adhesions in a patient with a history of abdominal surgery. During balloon-assisted enteroscopy, the small bowel was fixed and difficult to advance. The mucosa was normal. However, the lumen was shrunken, and the bowel did not distend when air was insufflated.

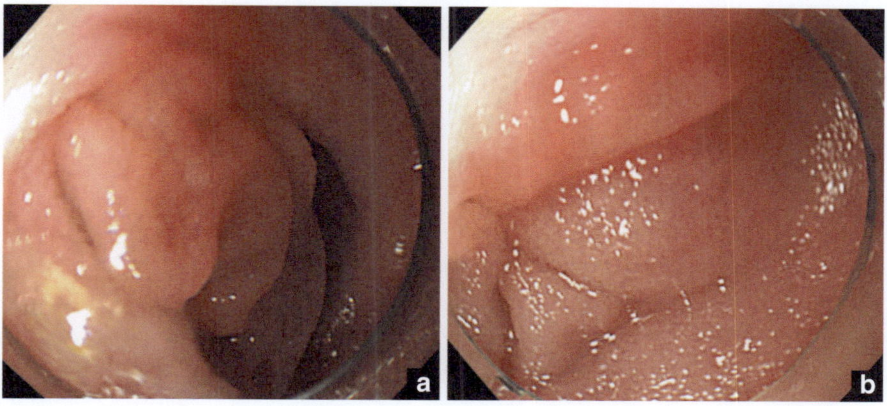

References

1. Hong SN, Kim ER, Ye BD, Jang HJ, Jeon SR, et al. Indications, diagnostic yield, and complication rate of balloon-assisted enteroscopy (BAE) during the first decade of its use in Korea. Dig Endosc. 2016;28(4):443–9. https://doi.org/10.1111/den.12593.
2. Hong YS, Woo YS, Park G, Lee K, Kang SH, et al. Endoscopic findings of enteropathy-associated T-cell lymphoma type II: a case series. Gut Liver. 2016;10(1):147–51. https://doi.org/10.5009/gnl14457.
3. Yamamoto H, Sakamoto H, Kumagai H, Abe T, Ishiguro S, et al. Clinical guidelines for diagnosis and Management of Peutz-Jeghers Syndrome in children and adults. Digestion. 2023;104(5):335–47. https://doi.org/10.1159/000529799.
4. Na JE, Kim HS, Hong SN, Song KD, Kim JE, et al. Comparison of an endoscopic scoring system and the simplified magnetic resonance index of activity in patients with small bowel Crohn's disease. Gut Liver. 2024;18(1):97–105. https://doi.org/10.5009/gnl220422. Epub 2023 Apr 4. PMID: 37013455; PMCID: PMC10791503
5. Hong SN, Kim JE, Kim ER, Chang DK, Kim YH. Enteroscopic balloon dilation in small bowel Stricturing Crohn's disease: long-term outcomes and risk factors for surgery in a single-Center prospective observational study. United European Gastroenterol J. 2025. Epub ahead of print; https://doi.org/10.1002/ueg2.12775.
6. Yano T, Yamamoto H, Sunada K, Miyata T, Iwamoto M, et al. Endoscopic classification of vascular lesions of the small intestine (with videos). Gastrointest Endosc. 2008;67(1):169–72. https://doi.org/10.1016/j.gie.2007.08.005.
7. Hong SN, Jang HJ, Ye BD, Jeon SR, Im JP, et al. Diagnosis of bleeding Meckel's diverticulum in adults. PLoS One. 2016;11(9):e0162615. https://doi.org/10.1371/journal.pone.0162615.

MIX
Papier aus verantwortungsvollen Quellen
Paper from responsible sources
FSC® C105338

If you have any concerns about our products,
you can contact us on
ProductSafety@springernature.com

In case Publisher is established outside the EU,
the EU authorized representative is:
Springer Nature Customer Service Center GmbH
Europaplatz 3, 69115 Heidelberg, Germany

Printed by Libri Plureos GmbH
in Hamburg, Germany